FIRST AID
— FOR —
CHILDREN
FAST

IN ASSOCIATION WITH THE

British Red Cross

FIRST AID
— FOR —
CHILDREN
FAST

Chief Medical Adviser: British Red Cross
Sir Cameron Moffat

Foreword by
Diana, Princess of Wales

DK

DORLING KINDERSLEY
London · New York · Sydney · Moscow

A DORLING KINDERSLEY BOOK

Project Editor
Caroline Greene

Senior Art Editor
Jane Bull

Managing Editor
Jemima Dunne

Managing Art Editor
Tina Vaughan

DTP Designer
Karen Ruane

Production
Maryann Rogers

Photography
Andy Crawford
Steve Gorton

First published in Great Britain in 1994
by Dorling Kindersley Limited,
9 Henrietta Street, London WC2E 8PS
Reprinted 1994, 1995, 1996, 1997

Visit us on the World Wide Web at
http://www.dk.com

A CIP catalogue record for this book is available from the British Library

ISBN 0 7513 0138 8

Reproduced in Italy by GRB Editrice, Verona
Printed and bound in Great Britain by
Butler & Tanner Ltd, Frome and London

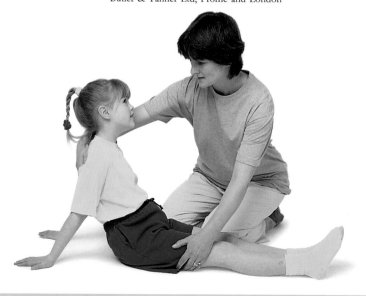

FOREWORD

Although the British Red Cross Society is perhaps best known as an agency that is quick to bring relief to those stricken by war, famine or natural disaster abroad, I have always been enormously impressed by its practical first aid training programmes at home.

All families can now benefit from this latest support to the Society's training programmes. As a parent I can think of nothing more precious than the health and safety of our children. *First Aid for Children Fast* is not a real substitute for the practical first aid training that is recommended for those entrusted with the care of children. It is, however, a clear and easy-to-use manual which I hope will give a happier ending to many every-day mishaps.

Diana.

Diana, Princess of Wales

Former Vice President of the British Red Cross

CONTENTS

INTRODUCTION

This book has been compiled primarily for parents but also for others – grandparents, teachers, child-minders, babysitters, playgroup leaders – who may regularly, or even occasionally, find themselves in charge of infants and children.

The content has been set out in a clear and logical way and the information presented largely in pictorial form using simple words and captions to make it very easy to follow and to understand. The First Aid methods and techniques described are in accordance with accepted modern practice and are in harmony with guidelines set out by the Paediatric Life Support Group of the European Resuscitation Council.

Emergencies are by their very nature unexpected events and require a prompt and proper response. If you follow the advice and guidance given in this book you will undoubtedly be able to give early and effective help whenever it is needed. You should be aware however that First Aid is essentially a practical skill and your confidence and effectiveness will be greatly enhanced by expert training in a practical setting. The British Red Cross has Branches and Centres throughout the country and regularly runs a wide variety of First Aid Courses, some exclusively concerned with First Aid for infants and children. You can find out more about these courses by ringing your local Red Cross – the number will be in your phone book – who will be very pleased to hear from you.

Giving First Aid – coping with the emergency and doing the right thing early and effectively – can be straightforward but it can also be stressful, sometimes distasteful (especially if the child is not your own), and even dangerous. It is important that you remain in control of your feelings and avoid any tendency to rash action which could result in additional harm to an injured child or to yourself. You cannot give effective help if you yourself become a casualty so you must always take a little time to think before you act. This book is intended to help you to do the right thing at the right time – safely and effectively.

Sir Cameron Moffat
Chief Medical Adviser: British Red Cross

How to use this book

This book covers first aid treatment for everything from minor cuts and grazes to resuscitation. For every condition a series of photographs shows you exactly what to do in an emergency. Key pieces of information are indicated on the photographs and supplementary advice can be found alongside in the step-by-step text.

The injuries are organised by type, in sections such as Wounds and Bleeding and Bites and Stings. However, in an emergency, the thumbnail index on the back cover will direct you straight to the relevant page.

There are also sections such as Action in an Emergency and Bandages and Dressings, that contain information for general reference.

Key signs and symptoms help you to recognise the conditions

Clear photographs illustrate every step of treatment

Annotations highlight essential action

The quick reference index on the back cover gives instant access to major first aid emergencies

Symbols highlight the action necessary for further medical attention

Cross-references direct you to other pages where information is given about associated injuries

Guide to the symbols
The following symbols and instructions appear if your child needs further medical attention:

✆ CALL A DOCTOR
(Telephone for further advice.)

✚ TAKE YOUR CHILD TO HOSPITAL
(Your child needs to be seen in the Accident and Emergency department.)

☎ CALL AN AMBULANCE
(Your child needs urgent medical attention and is best transported by ambulance to hospital.)

9

ACTION IN AN EMERGENCY

**In any emergency, particularly one involving children,
it is important to keep calm and act logically. Remember four steps:**

1 Assess the situation

- What happened?
- How did it happen?
- Is there more than one injured child?
- Is there any continuing danger?
- Is there anyone who can help?
- Do I need an ambulance?

2 Think of safety

- Do not risk injuring yourself – you cannot help if you become a casualty
- Remove any source of danger from your child
- Move your child only if you must and do so very carefully

3 Treat serious injuries first

In children, there are two conditions that immediately threaten life:

- *Serious bleeding* – this is usually obvious and can be brought under control (see BLEEDING p.46)
- *Inability to breathe* (see ABC OF RESUSCITATION p.14)

If more than one child is injured go quickly to the quiet one – he may be unconscious

4 Get help

Shout for help early – ask others to: • Make the area safe
- Call a doctor or an ambulance • Help with first aid
- Move a child to safety, if necessary

Telephoning for help

When you call the emergency services, ask for an ambulance and give the following information:

- Your telephone number
- The location of the accident
- The type of accident
- The number, sex, and age of the casualties
- Details about their condition
- Details of any hazards such as gas, power line damage, or fog

10

FIRE

Have an escape plan

Before an emergency happens, decide:
- *How would you get out of each room?*
- *How do you help babies and small children?*
- *Where will you meet when you've escaped?*

CHIP PAN FIRE • *Turn off stove or hob* • *Cover pan with lid, wet tea towel, or fire blanket – leave this on for half an hour* • *DO NOT throw water over the flames* • *If not under control, close the door, call the fire brigade, get everyone out of the house*

Escaping from a fire

1 Feel the door. If the door is cool, leave the room. If it is hot, see opposite.

REMEMBER • *Carry out babies and toddlers* • *Children over six should look after only themselves when escaping – don't ask them to do anything else.*
- *Close all doors behind you*
- *Meet outside your house*
- *NEVER go back inside* • *Phone for help from somewhere else*

2 If the door is hot, don't open it. Go to the window.

SHUT the door behind you

IF you have to escape through the window, slide your child out, hang onto him, then ask him to drop to the ground. Slide out yourself, hang from the ledge, then drop. If you have to break the glass first, put a blanket over the frame before escaping.

LEAVE quickly
DO NOT GO BACK

PLACE blanket to keep smoke out

KEEP children low, where air is clearest

OPEN window, call for help

Clothing on fire

If no water is available

Wrap the child tightly in a coat or blanket (not nylon or cellular), or other heavy fabric and lay him on the ground to stifle the flames.

If water is available

Lay the child down with the burning side uppermost and douse the child with water or other non-flammable liquid.

DO NOT *let the child run about in a panic; rapid movement will fan the flames.*
DO NOT *roll the child along the ground, or flames will spread.*

IF your own clothes catch fire, wrap yourself up in heavy material and lie down.

ELECTRICAL INJURY

If an electrical current passes through a child's body, it may cause the breathing and even the heart to stop. The current may cause burns both where it enters and leaves the body. Alternating current causes muscle spasms that can prevent a child letting go of an electric cable.

CONTACT *with high-voltage current, found in power lines and overhead cables, is usually fatal for a child. Severe burns result and the child may be thrown some distance from the point of contact.* **NEVER** *approach the injured child unless you are told officially that the power has been cut off, or you will be in danger from "arcing", or "jumping", high-voltage electricity.*

Low-voltage current

Children are at risk of suffering an electric shock if they play with electrical sockets or flex, or if they bring water into contact with an electrical appliance.

IF *the child seems unharmed, make him rest and observe his condition.* ℂ CALL A DOCTOR

1 Break the contact by switching off the current at the mains.

2 If you cannot switch off the current, stand on dry insulating material such as telephone books, or a wooden box. Use a wooden broom handle or chair to push the child's limbs away from the source.

IF *the child loses consciousness, assess his condition (see* UNCONSCIOUS BABY *p. 16;* CHILD *p. 22). Cool any burns with cold water (see* ELECTRICAL BURNS *p. 62). Be prepared to resuscitate. If breathing, place him in the* RECOVERY POSITION.

DO NOT *touch the child's skin with your hands. Pull at his clothes only as a last resort.*

STAND on insulating material

PUSH the source away

3 Without touching the child, wrap a dry towel around his feet and pull him away from the source.

☎ CALL AN AMBULANCE

WRAP a dry towel around his feet. Pull him away

DROWNING

Babies and young children can drown quickly if they slip into a pool or pond or are left unattended in a bath. Even 2.5cm (1in) of water is enough to cover a baby's nose and mouth if she falls forwards.

A CHILD *may get into difficulty in open water especially if it is turbulent or very cold. Rescue him quickly. Try to reach him from the shore or bank with your hand, or with a stick. Get him dry and warm as quickly as possible (see also HYPOTHERMIA p.94).*

1 Lift your child out of the water. Carry her with her head lower than her chest to reduce the risk of inhaling water.

KEEP her head lower than her chest

2 ✚ TAKE YOUR CHILD TO HOSPITAL, even if she seems recovered, as she may have inhaled water, causing lung damage.

The unconscious child

OPEN airway

CHECK for breathing

CHECK his pulse

PLACE in the recovery position if breathing

Remove any wet clothing and cover him with a dry towel or blanket. Assess his condition (see UNCONSCIOUS BABY p.16; CHILD p.22). Be prepared to resuscitate. If breathing, place him in the RECOVERY POSITION.

☎ CALL AN AMBULANCE

WATER *in the lungs and the effects of cold can increase resistance to artificial ventilation so you may need to breathe more firmly and more slowly to get the chest to rise.*

13

ABC OF RESUSCITATION

A baby or child who stops breathing will become unconscious because no oxygen reaches the brain. Lack of oxygen also causes the heartbeat to slow down until it stops altogether. If your child is unconscious and stops breathing, you need to clear the airway and breathe into the lungs (Artificial Ventilation). If the heartbeat has stopped or, in a baby, is very slow you need to drive blood to the brain with chest compressions. This combination of Artificial Ventilation and chest compressions is Cardiopulmonary Resuscitation (CPR).

FOR *a-step-by-step guide to* RESUSCITATING A BABY *see p.16.* **FOR** *a step-by-step guide to* RESUSCITATING A CHILD *see p.22*

ASSESS your baby and act on your findings

ASSESS your child and act on your findings

14

A is for airway

You need to open the air passage, or airway. Look for and remove any obstruction in the mouth. Tilt the head and lift the chin to bring the tongue away from the back of the throat.

For a baby

For a child

Blocked airway head not tilted

TONGUE fallen back

BLOCKED airway

Unblocked airway head tilted

TONGUE forward

UNBLOCKED airway

.**TILT** the head only slightly

TILT the head back to clear the airway

B is for breathing

For a baby

If your child is not breathing after the airway is open, you can blow your expired air into the lungs to get oxygen into the child's blood.

For a child

HOLD the nose and blow into the mouth

BREATHE gently into the mouth and nose until the chest rises

C is for circulation

For a baby

If your child's heart has stopped and there is no pulse, or if your baby's pulse is very slow, giving chest compressions will drive blood through the heart and around the body. This is always combined with Artificial Ventilation. The combination of techniques is known as CPR – Cardiopulmonary Resuscitation.

For a child

CHEST COMPRESSIONS are given with two fingers

CHEST COMPRESSIONS are given with one hand only

15

Assessing the situation

For a baby you need to discover three things:

1 Is the baby conscious?

2 Is breathing present?

3 Is there a pulse? Is it very slow?

Before you rush to help a baby or child, you must decide whether there is any continuing danger (such as fire, fumes, electricity, or loose masonry) to the child or to yourself. You cannot help if you become a casualty. Shout for help if there is someone within earshot. Always try to remove the danger from the child and move an injured child only if you must.

For a child you need to discover three things:

1 Is the child conscious?

2 Is breathing present?

3 Is there a pulse?

UNCONSCIOUS BABY

Assess your baby's condition.

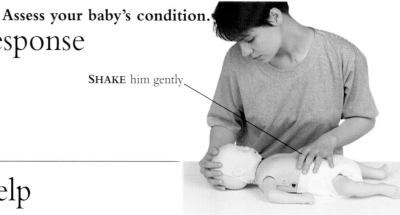

1 Check for response

- Shake your baby gently
- Call his name
- Pinch his skin

SHAKE him gently

2 Shout for help

3 Open the airway

- Remove any obvious obstruction from mouth
- Use one finger to lift the chin
- Tilt the head back only slightly

LOOK in mouth

LIFT chin with one finger

TILT head back very slightly

4 Check for breathing

- Listen for sounds of breathing
- Feel for breath on your cheek
- Look along the chest for movement
- Check for five seconds before deciding breathing is absent

LISTEN for breathing

LOOK for chest movement

FEEL for breath on your cheek

IF NOT *breathing, give five breaths of artificial ventilation (see p.18)*

PUT your mouth over baby's mouth and nose

5 Check for pulse

- Place your thumb on the outside of the arm midway between shoulder and elbow
- Use two fingers to feel for a pulse on the inner side of the arm, pressing gently towards the bone
- Feel for five seconds before deciding pulse is absent (a baby's normal pulse is about 120 beats a minute)

CHECK for a pulse on the inner side of upper arm

16

6 Act on your findings

Baby unconscious, breathing and pulse present

1 Treat any life-threatening injuries such as burns (p.60) or bleeding (p.46).

2 Cradle your baby in your arms with his head tilted.

3 CALL AN AMBULANCE
If you have no helper, take your baby with you to the telephone.

4 Keep your baby in your arms until help arrives.

Not breathing but good pulse present

1 Give about 20 breaths of mouth-to-mouth-and-nose ventilation for one minute. See overleaf.

2 CALL AN AMBULANCE
If you have no helper, take your baby with you to the telephone.

3 Continue giving mouth-to-mouth-and-nose ventilations.

4 Check for pulse every minute (after every 20 breaths).

Not breathing, pulse absent or very slow (less than 60 beats per minute)

1 Give Cardiopulmonary Resuscitation (CPR) – five chest compressions followed by one breath of mouth-to-mouth-and-nose artificial ventilation – repeated for one minute (see p.20).

2 CALL AN AMBULANCE
If you have no helper, take your baby with you to the telephone.

3 Continue giving Cardiopulmonary Resuscitation (CPR) until help arrives.

17

ARTIFICIAL VENTILATION: BABY

To be used for an unconscious baby who is not breathing but has a good pulse (faster than 60 beats per minute). See p.16.

RESUSCITATION SUMMARY

UNCONSCIOUS BABY

AIRWAY OPEN

NO BREATHING

GIVE 5 BREATHS OF **ARTIFICIAL VENTILATION**

GOOD PULSE PRESENT

GIVE **ARTIFICIAL VENTILATION** FOR 1 MINUTE

GOOD PULSE PRESENT

☎ CALL AN AMBULANCE

CONTINUE **ARTIFICIAL VENTILATION** UNTIL HELP ARRIVES

18

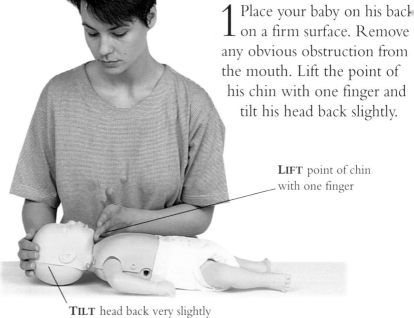

1 Place your baby on his back on a firm surface. Remove any obvious obstruction from the mouth. Lift the point of his chin with one finger and tilt his head back slightly.

LIFT point of chin with one finger

TILT head back very slightly

2 Seal your lips tightly around your baby's mouth and nose. Breathe gently into the lungs until the chest rises.

BREATHE into the baby's mouth and nose

LET the chest rise

REMOVE your mouth

3 Remove your lips and let the chest fall back.

IF *your baby's chest does not rise, check the mouth again. Do not put a finger down the throat unless you see an obstruction.*

WATCH the chest fall back

GIVE one breath every three seconds

WATCH chest fall after each breath

4 Continue to ventilate for one minute, aiming for one complete breath every three seconds (a rate of 20 breaths per minute).

CHECK the pulse on his upper arm

5 Stop and check that the pulse is still good (see p.16). If it becomes very slow or is absent, start Cardiopulmonary Resuscitation, or CPR (see overleaf).

6 ☎ CALL AN AMBULANCE
If you have no helper, take your baby with you to the telephone.

7 Continue artificial ventilation until help arrives. Check the arm pulse every minute. If it becomes very slow or is absent, start CPR (see overleaf).

GIVE one breath every three seconds

WATCH chest fall after each breath

CHECK his pulse every minute

19

CPR ^(CARDIOPULMONARY RESUSCITATION) : BABY

To be used for an unconscious baby who is not breathing and has no pulse or a very slow pulse of less than 60 beats per minute. See p.16.

RESUSCITATION SUMMARY

UNCONSCIOUS BABY

AIRWAY OPEN

NO BREATHING

GIVE 5 BREATHS OF ARTIFICIAL VENTILATION, See P.18

NO PULSE OR VERY SLOW PULSE

CPR – 5 CHEST COMPRESSIONS, 1 BREATH OF ARTIFICIAL VENTILATION – REPEATED FOR 1 MINUTE

☎ CALL AN AMBULANCE

CONTINUE **CPR** UNTIL HELP ARRIVES

1 Place your baby on a firm surface. Place the tips of two fingers on the lower breastbone just below the nipple line.

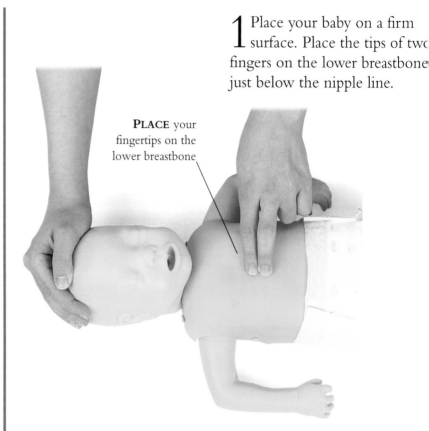

PLACE your fingertips on the lower breastbone

PRESS down to a depth of 2cm

2 Press down sharply at this point to a depth of 2cm. Do this five times within three seconds.

GIVE five compressions in three seconds

3 Give one full breath of artificial ventilation (see p.18).

GIVE one mouth-to-mouth-and-nose breath

Repeat steps 2 and 3 for one minute (ten cycles)

GIVE five chest compressions

4 Continue the cycles of five chest compressions to one breath for one minute (ten cycles).

FOLLOW with one breath

21

Repeat CPR cycles until help arrives

5 ☎ CALL AN AMBULANCE
If you have no helper, take your baby with you to the telephone.

6 Continue giving CPR – five chest compressions followed by one breath of artificial ventilation – until the ambulance arrives.

GIVE five chest compressions

FOLLOW with one breath

UNCONSCIOUS CHILD

Assess your child's condition.

1 Check for response
- Shake her gently
- Call her name
- Pinch her skin

SHAKE her gently

2 Shout for help

3 Open the airway
- Look in the mouth and remove any obstruction
- Place two fingers under the chin and lift the jaw
- Place other hand on the forehead and tilt the head back

LOOK in the mouth

PLACE tw fingers unde chin and li

TILT head back

4 Check for breathing
- Listen for sounds of breathing
- Feel for breath on your cheek
- Look along the chest for movement
- Check for five seconds before deciding if breathing is absent

IF NOT *breathing, give five breaths of artificial ventilation (see p.26)*

PUT your mouth over child's mouth and breathe

LISTEN f breathing

LOOK for chest movements

FEEL for breath on your cheek

5 Check for pulse
- Keep the head tilted
- Feel for the large muscle at the side of the neck
- Slide two fingers into the groove in front of this muscle
- Press lightly backwards

CHECK for a pulse at her neck

22

6 Act on your findings

Child unconscious, breathing and pulse present

1 Treat any life-threatening injuries such as burns (see p.60) or bleeding (see p.46).

2 Place her in the recovery position (see overleaf).

3 ☎ CALL AN AMBULANCE
Do not leave her alone. Keep a check on her breathing and be prepared to resuscitate.

Not breathing but pulse present

1 Give about 20 breaths of mouth-to-mouth ventilation for one minute (see p.26).

2 ☎ CALL AN AMBULANCE

3 Continue giving mouth-to-mouth ventilations.

4 Check for pulse every minute (after every 20 breaths).

Not breathing, no pulse

1 Give Cardiopulmonary Resuscitation (CPR) – five chest compressions followed by one breath of mouth-to-mouth artificial ventilation – repeated for one minute (see p.28).

2 ☎ CALL AN AMBULANCE

3 Continue Cardiopulmonary Resuscitation (CPR) until help arrives.

23

RECOVERY POSITION

Put your child in this position if she is unconscious, breathing and has a pulse
(see p.22), to prevent her choking on her tongue or vomit.

TILT her head back

LIFT her chin forward

MAKE sure her airway is clear

STRAIGHTEN her legs

BEND arm nearest to you at a right angle

PLACE back of her hand on the ground

MOVE furthest arm across her chest and bend it

PLACE back of her hand against her cheek

1 Kneel beside your child. Ti
her head back and lift her
chin forward. This keeps her a
passages open while you put
her in the recovery position.

IF *you suspect BACK AND NECK
INJURIES, see pp. 73–74.*

BE *very careful if you think there is a
broken bone. Move her so the injured
side is uppermost. See BONE, JOINT
AND MUSCLE INJURIES, pp. 76–84.*

2 If necessary, straighten
her legs. Bend the arm
nearest to you so that it make
a right angle and lay it on the
ground, with the palm of the
hand upward.

3 Bring her
other arm
across her chest.
Hold the back of her hand
against her opposite cheek.

24

PLACE her foot flat on ground

CLASP under thigh of outside leg and bend at knee

KEEP this leg straight

4 Use your free hand to clasp gently under the thigh furthest from you. Carefully pull the knee up to bend the leg, leaving the foot flat on the ground.

SUPPORT her hand against her cheek

ROLL her over onto her side by pulling bent leg towards you

KEEP her hand against her cheek

USE your knees to stop her rolling onto her front

5 Keep your child's hand against her cheek to support her head. At the same time, pull on the thigh of the bent leg to roll her towards you and onto her side.

IF *your child is already lying on her side or is on her front, you will need to adapt the steps when placing her in the recovery position.*

CHECK *your child's breathing and pulse frequently while you are waiting for help to arrive.*

ADJUST hand under her cheek

TILT head back again to make sure airway is still open

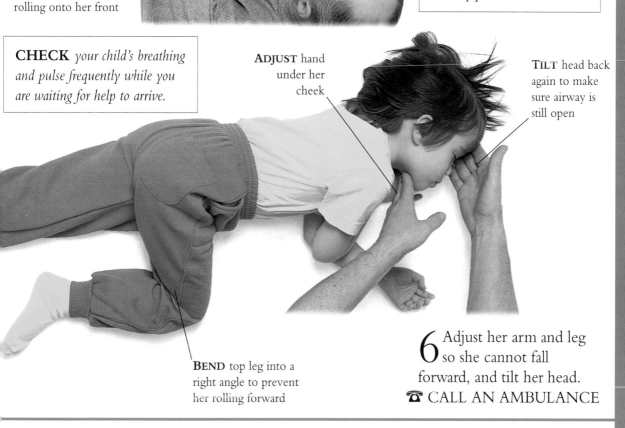

BEND top leg into a right angle to prevent her rolling forward

6 Adjust her arm and leg so she cannot fall forward, and tilt her head.
☎ CALL AN AMBULANCE

25

ARTIFICIAL VENTILATION: CHILI

**If an unconscious child is not breathing but still has a pulse,
you must give mouth-to-mouth ventilation. See p.22.**

**RESUSCITATION
SUMMARY**

UNCONSCIOUS CHILD

AIRWAY OPEN

NO BREATHING

GIVE 5 BREATHS OF
**ARTIFICIAL
VENTILATION**

PULSE PRESENT

GIVE
**ARTIFICIAL
VENTILATION**
FOR 1 MINUTE

PULSE PRESENT

☎ CALL AN
AMBULANCE

CONTINUE
**ARTIFICIAL
VENTILATION**
UNTIL HELP
ARRIVES

1 Place your child on her
 back on a firm surface.
Remove any obvious
obstruction from her
mouth. Lift the point of her
chin using two fingers
and tilt her head back.

LIFT point of chin
with two fingers

TILT the
head back

PINCH
nostrils
closed

2 Pinch her nostrils
 closed. Seal your lips
round her open mouth.
Breathe into the lungs until
you see the chest rise.

SEAL your lips
around her mouth

BREATHE until the chest rises

26

REMOVE
your
mouth

KEEP
nostrils
pinched

3 Remove your mouth and let the chest fall. Keep the nostrils pinched.

> **IF** *your child's chest does not rise, check the mouth again. Do not put your fingers blindly down the throat unless you see an obstruction.*

WATCH the chest fall

GIVE one breath every three seconds

WATCH the chest fall

4 Continue to ventilate for one minute, aiming for a complete breath every three seconds (a rate of 20 per minute), or slightly slower in an older child.

CHECK the pulse at her neck

5 Stop and check that the neck pulse is still present (see p.22). If it is absent, start Cardiopulmonary Resuscitation, or CPR (see overleaf).

6 ☎ CALL AN AMBULANCE

7 Continue artificial ventilation until help arrives. Check the neck pulse every minute and if it is absent, begin CPR.

GIVE one breath every three seconds

WATCH the chest fall after each breath

CHECK her pulse every minute

27

CPR (CARDIOPULMONARY RESUSCITATION) : CHILD

To be used when an unconscious child is not breathing and has no pulse in the neck. See p.22. Give CPR for a full minute before you call an ambulance.

RESUSCITATION SUMMARY

UNCONSCIOUS CHILD

AIRWAY OPEN

NO BREATHING

GIVE 5 BREATHS OF ARTIFICIAL VENTILATION, See P.26

NO PULSE

CPR – 5 CHEST COMPRESSIONS, 1 BREATH OF ARTIFICIAL VENTILATION, REPEATED FOR 1 MINUTE

☎ CALL AN AMBULANCE

CONTINUE **CPR** UNTIL HELP ARRIVES

FEEL where the ribs meet and place index finger on bone above

PUT middle finger on tip of breastbone

1 Place your child on her back on a firm surface. Find the point where the ribs meet in the middle line. Place your middle finger on the tip of the breastbone and your index finger on the bone above it.

SLIDE other hand along breastbone to meet fingers

2 Slide the heel of your other hand down the breastbone to meet your fingers.

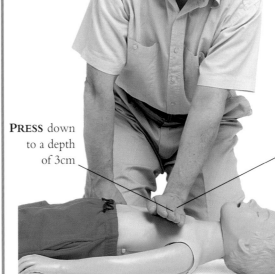

3 Using the heel of the top hand only, press down sharply at this point to a depth of 3cm. Do this five times within three seconds.

PRESS down to a depth of 3cm

COMPRESS chest five times in three seconds

GIVE one mouth-to-mouth breath

4 Give one full breath of artificial ventilation (see p.26).

WATCH chest fall

Repeat steps 3 and 4 for one minute (ten cycles)

GIVE five chest compressions

5 Continue the cycles of five chest compressions to one breath for one minute (ten cycles).

FOLLOW with one breath

Repeat CPR cycles until help arrives

GIVE five chest compressions

FOLLOW with one breath

6 ☎ CALL AN AMBULANCE

DO NOT *stop to make pulse checks unless there are clear signs of life. If pulse and breathing return, place your child in the* RECOVERY POSITION *(see p.24) and watch her carefully until the ambulance arrives.*

7 Continue giving CPR – five chest compressions followed by one breath of artificial ventilation – until the ambulance arrives.

SHOCK

Recognising shock This develops from the early signs of • *Pale, cold, and sweaty skin, tinged with grey* • *A rapid pulse becoming weaker* • *Shallow, fast breathing,* to the later signs of • *Restlessness, yawning, and sighing* • *Thirst* • *Loss of consciousness*

> **THE** *most likely cause of shock in a child is serious BLEEDING, see p.46, or a SEVERE BURN OR SCALD, see p.60. These injuries must be treated without delay.*

> **DO NOT** *give your child anything to drink or eat. If he is thirsty, moisten his lips with water.*

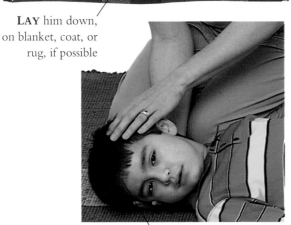

MOVE your child as little as possible

LAY him down, on blanket, coat, or rug, if possible

KEEP his head flat on floor and turn it to one side

1 Lay your child down flat. Keep his head low as this improves the blood supply to the brain. Turn his head to one side and reassure him. Treat any injury.

☎ CALL AN AMBULANCE

2 Carefully raise your child's legs and support them with pillows, on a chair, or on a pile of books padded with a cushion.

KEEP his head lower than his chest

CONTINUE to reassure him

RAISE his legs high above heart level

30

3 To make breathing easier, loosen any fastenings or tight clothing at his neck, chest, or waist.

LOOSEN any tight clothing

GIVE constant reassurance

OBSERVE his breathing rate and skin colour

4 Put a blanket or coat over your child to protect him from cold. DO NOT give him a hot-water bottle or apply any other source of direct heat.

TRY NOT *to leave a child in shock unattended. If you can, send someone else to phone for the ambulance while you stay with him.*

KEEP checking his pulse

COVER him with a blanket to keep him warm

5 Keep reassuring your child. Encourage him to talk or answer questions. This will help you assess his condition. Note any changes and tell the ambulance attendant.

IF *he loses consciousness, assess his condition (see* UNCONSCIOUS BABY *p.16;* CHILD *p.22). Be prepared to resuscitate. If breathing, place him in the* RECOVERY POSITION.

FEBRILE CONVULSIONS

Young children under the age of four may develop these convulsions when they have an infection and a high temperature.

Recognising a convulsion • *He may be flushed and sweating with a very hot forehead* • *His eyes may roll upwards, be fixed or squinting* • *His face may look blue if he is holding his breath* • *He may stiffen and arch his back* • *His fists may clench*

COOL him by taking off his clothes and bedclothes

1 Undress him down to his nappy. Make sure there is plenty of fresh air in the room without it being cold.

2 Clear a space around him to protect him from injury. Sponge him with tepid water by starting at his head and working down his body. Do not let him get too cold.

SPONGE him with tepid water until temperature falls

COVER him with a sheet

ROLL him onto his side

3 When the child is cooled, convulsions will stop. Roll him onto his side and try to keep his head tilted back. Cover him with a light blanket or sheet and reassure him. If his temperature rises again, sponge him again.

℄ CALL A DOCTOR

IF *you can, place him in the RECOVERY POSITION (see p.24) once the convulsions have come to an end.*

EPILEPTIC CONVULSIONS

Recognising major epilepsy A fit progresses through the following stages: • *Sudden falling into unconsciousness, sometimes with a cry* • *Rigidity and arching of back* • *Breathing may cease* • *Jerking, movements* • *Froth or bubbles around the mouth, may be blood stained* • *Bladder or bowel control lost* • *Conscious within a few minutes* • *Dazed feeling* • *Deep sleep may follow*

Children with a history of epilepsy may have a card or bracelet alerting you to this. A child may have a minor fit before a major one. This can be recognised by a momentary "switching off", some facial twitching, or distracted movements such as lip-smacking. If this happens, reassure the child and arrange to see your doctor.

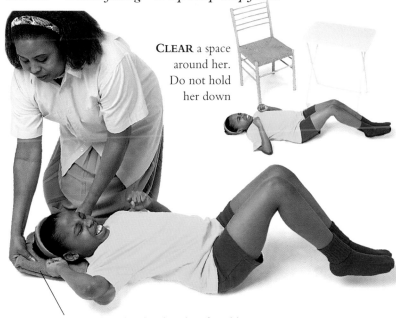

CLEAR a space around her. Do not hold her down

PROTECT her head with soft padding

1 If your child starts to fall, try to catch her and help her to the floor. Clear away objects that she may knock against. Put padding under or around her head. Do not hold her down or try to move her. Don't put anything in her mouth or give her anything to eat or drink.

33

Once the convulsions have stopped

OPEN airway

CHECK for breathing

CHECK her pulse

PLACE her in the recovery position if breathing

2 When her convulsions are over, she may be unconscious. Remove any padding, check the airway is open, and that breathing and pulse are present. If breathing, place her in the RECOVERY POSITION (see p.24). Stay with her until she is recovered. She may feel dazed and behave oddly, or she may sleep deeply.
Ⓒ CALL A DOCTOR

IF *your child has never had a fit before, if she fits, relaxes and fits again, or if she remains unconscious for more than ten minutes,*
☎ CALL AN AMBULANCE

DIABETIC EMERGENCY

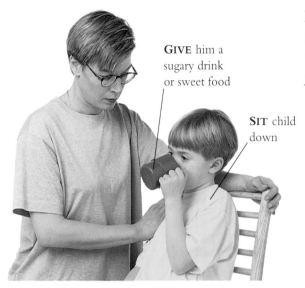

GIVE him a sugary drink or sweet food

SIT child down

Recognising low blood sugar • *Weakness or hunger* • *Confused or aggressive behaviour* • *Sweating* • *A very pale face* • *A strong, bounding pulse* • *Shallow breathing*

> *A child who is diabetic is likely to be on insulin. Even if he seems recovered, a doctor should be asked to check the insulin dosage.*

If he improves rapidly after a sweet drink or food, give him some more and let him rest. If he does not,
☎ CALL AN AMBULANCE

An unconscious child

OPEN airway

CHECK for breathing

CHECK her pulse

PLACE her in the recovery position if breathing

1 Open the airway and check that breathing and pulse are present.

> **IF** *your child is not breathing, be prepared to resuscitate (see* UNCONSCIOUS BABY *p.16;* CHILD *p.22).*

2 If she is breathing, place her in the RECOVERY POSITION (see p.24).

☎ CALL AN AMBULANCE

34

FAINT

PLACE her head between her knees

TELL her to take deep breaths

Recognising a faint • *A feeling of weakness, giddiness, and sickness* • *A very pale face* • *A brief loss of consciousness* • *A slow pulse*

1 Tell your child to sit down with her head between her knees. Alternatively, lay her down and raise her legs above the level of her heart, supporting them on a pile of cushions, pillows, or folded blankets.

LOOSEN any tight clothing

RAISE her legs to improve blood flow to her brain

COOL her by fanning her face

2 Check that there is no tight clothing around her neck, chest, and waist. Give her plenty of fresh air – open a window, if you are indoors. It may help to fan her face.

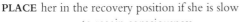

PLACE her in the recovery position if she is slow to regain consciousness

3 If your child does not regain consciousness, assess her condition (see UNCONSCIOUS BABY p.16; CHILD p.22). Be prepared to resuscitate. If breathing, place her in the RECOVERY POSITION.
☎ CALL AN AMBULANCE

35

CHOKING: BABY

SUMMARY

GIVE 5 SHARP
BACK SLAPS

GIVE 5 CHEST
THRUSTS

CHECK MOUTH

REPEAT CYCLE

5 BACK SLAPS
5 CHEST THRUSTS
CHECK MOUTH

until help arrives
or
obstruction clears

Recognising a choking child • *Breathing is obstructed* • *Face may turn blue* • *Trying to cry but making strange noises, or no sound*

1 Lay your baby face down with his head low along your forearm. Support his head and shoulders on your hand and give five sharp slaps between his shoulders.

> **DO NOT** *shake him or hold him upside down.*

LAY him along your forearm

KEEP his head low and support his chin

GIVE five sharp slaps on his back

2 If back slaps fail to clear the blockage turn him face up along your other arm. Place two fingers on the lower half of the breastbone and give five sharp downward thrusts. These act as artificial coughs.

TURN him onto his back

SUPPORT his head and keep it low

PLACE two fingers on breastbone, just below nipple line

GIVE five sharp downward thrusts

36

3 Look in his mouth. Put your finger on his tongue to clear the view. Do not put a finger down the throat unless you can see the obstruction to hook it out.

If the blockage hasn't cleared, ☎ CALL AN AMBULANCE

LOOK IN his mouth and remove any object you can see

Repeat cycle, following steps 1-3, until help arrives or the obstruction is cleared

GIVE five back slaps

GIVE five chest thrusts

CHECK mouth

IF *your baby loses consciousness, see UNCONSCIOUS BABY p.16. Be prepared to resuscitate.*

CHOKING: CHILD

SUMMARY

ENCOURAGE CHILD
TO COUGH

⬇

GIVE 5 BACK SLAPS

⬇

GIVE 5 CHEST THRUSTS
(artificial coughs)

⬇

CHECK MOUTH

⬇

GIVE 5 ABDOMINAL
THRUSTS

⬇

CHECK MOUTH

⬇

REPEAT CYCLE

give 5 back slaps
give 5 chest thrusts
check mouth
give 5 abdominal thrusts until help
arrives or obstruction clears

Recognising a choking child • *Sudden clutching at the throat* • *Child unable to speak or breathe* • *Face may go blue*

IF *she becomes unconscious at any stage, the throat may relax and she may be able to breathe. If she does not breathe, begin resuscitation (see p.22). Continue until help arrives.*

Choking in a small child You need to follow the same actions as for an older child, but you may find it easier to keep the child across your lap. Use less force for a very small child than for an older child.

1 Your child may be able to cough up on her own. Encourage her to do this, but do not waste time.

GET her to cough up if she can

2 Make her bend well forward. Give her five sharp slaps between the shoulder blades.

For small child

BEND her over your knees

GIVE her five sharp slaps between shoulder blades

For older child

BEND her well forward

GIVE her five sharp slaps between shoulder blades

38

For small child

SUPPORT her back on your thigh

GIVE five downwards thrusts

PLACE heel of your hand on lower breastbone

3 If back slaps fail, lay her on a firm surface. Lay an older child on the floor. Lay a small child over your knees, her back resting firmly on your thigh. Give chest thrusts: place heel of one hand over the lower breastbone. Thrust sharply downwards up to five times.

For older child

LAY her on the floor

PLACE heel of your hand on lower breastbone

GIVE five downwards thrusts

LOOK in the mouth

4 Look in her mouth. Use a finger on the tongue for a clear view. Remove any object you can see.

> **DO NOT** *put a finger blindly down the throat*

LOOK in the mouth

REMOVE any object you can see

CE heel of below **bs**

REMOVE any object you see

5 If the blockage has not cleared, give abdominal thrusts. Place the heel of one hand in the middle of the upper abdomen just below the rib cage and give five firm upward thrusts.

Check her mouth.

PLACE heel of hand below the ribs

GIVE five upward thrusts

HECK her mouth

GIVE five upward thrusts

☎ CALL AN AMBULANCE

CHECK her mouth

TURN her over

GIVE her five back slaps

Repeat the cycle until help arrives or blockage clears. Begin with back slaps again. Keep an older child on the floor. Keep a smaller child on your knees.

Then follow steps 3 – 5.

TURN her onto her side on the floor

GIVE her five back slaps

39

BREATH HOLDING

Recognising breath holding Only children under four years of age are likely to do this. • *Your child cries, breathes in but does not breathe out* • *He may go blue in the face and stiff* • *He may become unconscious momentarily*

Breath holding is the result of rage and frustration. Try to stay calm. Do not shake him or make a fuss. He will usually start breathing again spontaneously. If he loses consciousness, see UNCONSCIOUS BABY p.16; CHILD, p.22.

☎ CALL AN AMBULANCE

BLOW into his face

> **IF** *your baby holds his breath, blow in his face to start him breathing again.*

HICCUPS

TELL your child to sit quietly

URGE her to hold her breath for as long as possible

OR

An older child may be able to halt the attack by drinking from the wrong side of a cup.
IF *the hiccups go on for longer than a few hours,* ℂ CALL A DOCTOR, *as a long attack can be worrying, tiring, and painful.*

ASK her to hold a paper bag over her mouth and nose

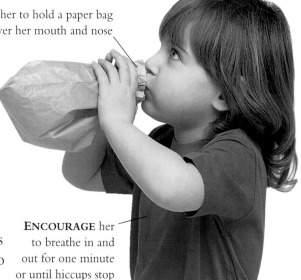

Tell your child to sit still and to hold her breath for as long as she can. Repeat this until the hiccups have gone.
OR
Hold a paper bag over her face so that she is re-breathing her own expired air. Get her to breathe in and out for about one minute.

ENCOURAGE her to breathe in and out for one minute or until hiccups stop

SUFFOCATION

This occurs when there is an obstruction over the mouth or nose, a weight on the child's chest or abdomen preventing normal breathing, or because the child is breathing in smoke- or fume-filled air.

REMOVE obstruction

1 Take away the obstruction as quickly as possible. This may restore breathing.

2 Open the airway. Place two fingers under the chin and lift the jaw. Place your hand on his forehead and tilt his head well back. Look and listen for breathing.

OPEN airway

CHECK for breathing

IF *he is not breathing, see* UNCONSCIOUS BABY *p.16;* CHILD *p.22. Be prepared to resuscitate.*

CHECK his pulse

3 If he is breathing, place him in the RECOVERY POSITION (see p.24). Continue to check his breathing and pulse rate.
☎ CALL AN AMBULANCE

PLACE him in the recovery position if breathing

41

STRANGULATION

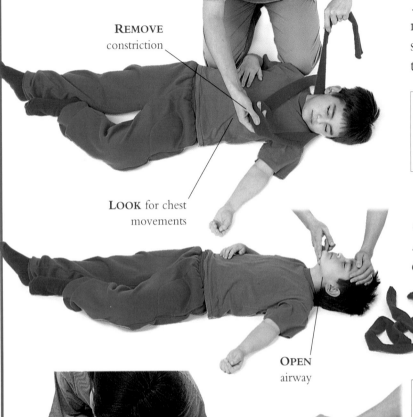

REMOVE constriction

LOOK for chest movements

OPEN airway

CHECK for breathing

CHECK his pulse

PLACE him in the recovery position if breathing

1 Remove the constriction from around your child's neck without delay. Use scissors or a knife if they are to hand.

> **IF** *the child is hanging, support the body while you remove the rope or cord.*

2 Open the airway. Place two fingers under the chin and lift the jaw. Place your hand on his forehead and tilt his head well back. Look and listen for breathing.

> **IF** *he is not breathing, see* UNCONSCIOUS BABY *p.16;* CHILD *p.22. Be prepared to resuscitate.*

3 If your child is breathing, place him in the RECOVERY POSITION (see p.24). Keep checking his breathing and pulse while you wait.
☎ CALL AN AMBULANCE

> **IF** *you suspect BACK OR NECK INJURIES, see pp.73-74.*

42

FUME INHALATION

Fume, gas, and smoke inhalation requires urgent medical attention.

☎ CALL AMBULANCE AND FIRE SERVICES

1 Carry your child away from the area of danger, without putting yourself at risk.

LOOK for chest movements

REMOVE your child into fresh air

> IF *your child has any* BURNS, *see p.60.*

2 Open the airway. Place two fingers under the chin and lift the jaw. At the same time, place your hand on her forehead and tilt her head well back.

43

3 Check for breathing. Feel for breath on your face and look for chest movements.

OPEN airway

CHECK for breathing

> IF *your child is not breathing, see* UNCONSCIOUS BABY *p.16;* CHILD *p.22. Be prepared to resuscitate.*

CHECK her pulse

4 If the child is breathing, place her in the RECOVERY POSITION (see p.24) while you wait for help to arrive. Continue to monitor her breathing and pulse rate.

PLACE her in the recovery position if breathing

CROUP

Recognising croup This usually occurs at night. It may be alarming, but usually passes quickly. • *Difficulty breathing, particularly inhaling* • *Short, barking cough* • *Crowing or whistling noise.* In a severe attack • *Evidence that the child is using muscles around the nose, neck, upper arms in his attempts to breathe* • *Blue-tinged skin*

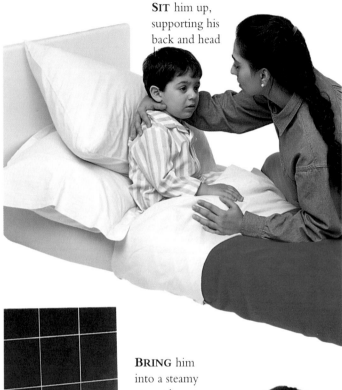

SIT him up, supporting his back and head

IF *the attack is severe and affects an older child, there is a slight risk that he is suffering a rare croup-like condition called epiglottitis. Suspect epiglottitis if your child has a high temperature and is sitting bolt upright, obviously in distress.*
☎ CALL AN AMBULANCE

1 Help your child to sit up in bed. Prop him up with pillows at his back and head and reassure him.

BRING him into a steamy atmosphere to ease his breathing

KEEP your child well clear of hot running water

2 Create a steamy atmosphere; run hot water into the bath or boil a kettle in an enclosed room. Try to get your child to relax enough to breathe in the steam.

IF *the attack is severe or prolonged,* ℂ CALL A DOCTOR.
Try to stay calm: if you panic this may alarm your child and worsen the attack.

44

ASTHMA

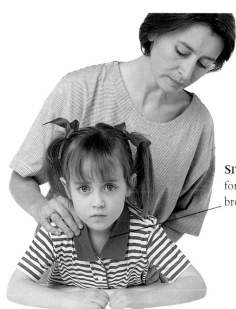

Recognising asthma • *Difficulty in breathing often accompanied by coughing* • *Wheezing on breathing out* • *Distress and anxiety* • *Tiredness from laboured breathing* • *Bluish tinge to face and lips*

SIT her forward to ease breathing

1 Ensure the room is well-ventilated and smoke-free.

> **IF** *it is a first attack,*
> ℭ CALL A DOCTOR.
> **IF** *the attack is severe or does not respond to medication,*
> ☎ CALL AN AMBULANCE.

OR

SIT her on your lap

2 Help your child to relax. Sit her down with her arms resting on a table or sit her on your lap. Reassure her as she will be frightened.

45

> **IF** *your child has special medication, use it early in any attack, see below.*

Taking medication

If your child has medication, let him use it. Follow the directions carefully. The attack should ease. If it does not, ☎ CALL AN AMBULANCE.

HELP him to use his inhaler, if he has one

Various types of medication are prescribed. Familiarise your child with his medication so that he knows how to use it when he has an attack.

BLEEDING

PRESS on wound

RAISE injured part

1 Press firmly on the wound to stop the bleeding. Press over a clean pad or handkerchief or put the palm of your hand directly on the wound. Raise the injured part above the level of the child's heart.

> **IF** *an object has become stuck in the wound, see* EMBEDDED OBJECT, *p. 48.*

LAY child down, keeping injured part high

CONTINUE pressing on wound

2 Lay your child down, with her head low (put a thin pad under her head for comfort), and keep the injured part raised above the heart. Keep pressing on the wound for up to ten minutes.

KEEP her head low – use a thin pad for comfort

BANDAGE a sterile dressing firmly but not too tightly in place, over the pad

3 Cover the wound with a sterile dressing that is larger than the wound. Bandage the dressing in place, still keeping the injured part raised. The bandage should be firm, but not so tight as to cut off the blood supply.

KEEP injured part raised

> **IF** *blood comes through the bandage, bandage another pad firmly on top.*

46

SUPPORT
injured part
in a raised
position

4 When the bleeding is under control, support the injury–for example, with an ELEVATION SLING (see p.111).

✚ TAKE YOUR CHILD TO HOSPITAL

> **IF** *the bleeding persists, follow the treatment for* SHOCK, *below.*
> ☎ CALL AN AMBULANCE

Shock

1 If the bleeding doesn't stop, raise her legs high and support them on cushions.

☎ CALL AN AMBULANCE

2 Loosen any tight clothing and cover her with a blanket to keep her warm. If she is thirsty, moisten her lips with water, but don't let her drink or eat. (For more on SHOCK, see pp.30–31.)

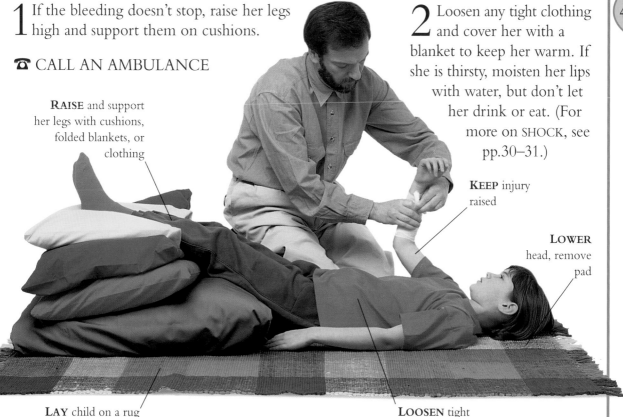

RAISE and support
her legs with cushions,
folded blankets, or
clothing

KEEP injury
raised

LOWER
head, remove
pad

LAY child on a rug
or blanket

LOOSEN tight
clothing

47

EMBEDDED OBJECT

APPLY pressure on either side of the wound

RAISE and support injured part

CONTINUE pressure on either side of wound

DO *not try to remove objects that are embedded in a wound as you may cause further damage and bleeding.*

1 Help your child to rest. Apply pressure on either side of the object and raise the injured part above the level of your child's heart.

DRAPE a piece of gauze over wound

2 Place a piece of gauze over the wound and object to minimise the risk of infection.

3 Use spare bandage rolls to build up padding to the same height as the embedded object.

PLACE padding around the object

BANDAGE over padding

4 Secure the padding by bandaging over it, being careful not to press on the embedded object.
+ TAKE YOUR CHILD TO HOSPITAL

Bandaging around larger objects

PROTECT object with pads

BANDAGE around object

IF *the object is very big, build padding around it and bandage above and below object.*

48

CUTS AND GRAZES

SIT child down

WASH graze

1 Sit your child down and gently wash the graze with soap and water using a gauze pad or a very soft brush.

REMOVE any dirt

2 Try to remove any particles of dirt or gravel. This may cause a little fresh bleeding.

IF *you cannot remove embedded particles of dirt,*
✚ TAKE YOUR CHILD TO HOSPITAL
Treatment will prevent a tattoo effect forming when the wound heals.

49

PRESS clean pad on graze

3 Apply pressure with a clean pad to stop bleeding.

PROTECT graze with a plaster

4 Dress the cut or graze with a plaster that has a pad large enough to cover the wound and the area around it.

DO NOT *cover cuts with cotton wool, or any fluffy material that may stick to the wound and delay healing.*

INFECTED WOUND

Recognising an infected wound • *Increasing pain and soreness* • *Swelling, redness, and a feeling of heat around the injury* • *Pus within, or oozing from, the wound* • *Swelling and tenderness of glands in the neck, armpit, or groin* • *Faint red trails on the skin leading to these glands.* When infection is advanced • *Feverish signs of sweating, thirst, shivering, and lethargy*

COVER wound with a clean pad

BANDAGE it in place

1 Cover the wound with a clean non-fluffy pad or sterile dressing and then bandage it in place.

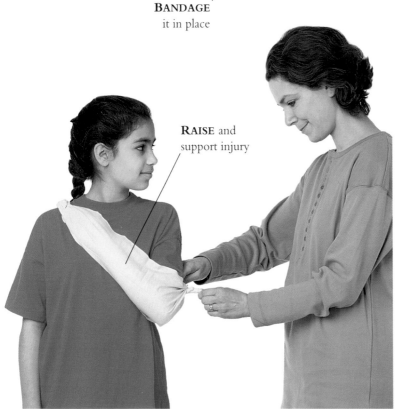

RAISE and support injury

2 Raise and support the infected wound, for example with an ELEVATION SLING (see p.111).

℡ CALL A DOCTOR

TETANUS *is a dangerous infection that is carried in the air or in the soil. Once present in a wound tetanus germs release toxins (poisons) into the nervous system. It is best prevented through vaccination. Babies receive this as part of their immunisation programme and a booster is given before starting school.*

50

BLISTERS

CLEAN blister with soap and water

1 Clean the blister thoroughly with soap and water. Rinse it with clean water.

IF *the blister has been caused by a burn, see BURNS AND SCALDS, p.60.*

PAT dry with clean pad

2 Thoroughly dry the blister and the surrounding skin. Pat it gently with a clean pad or paper tissues.

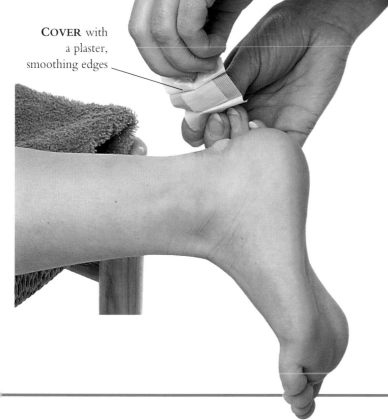

COVER with a plaster, smoothing edges

3 Cover the blister with a plaster. Make sure it is smooth. The plaster needs to have a pad large enough to cover the whole blister.

IF *the blister is very large, cover it with a clean, non-fluffy dressing and hold it in place with adhesive tape or a bandage. Never deliberately break a blister as this can cause it to become infected.*

51

EYE WOUND

LAY the child down

KEEP his head supported

TELL him to keep both eyes still

FOR *FOREIGN BODY IN THE EYE see p.86.*
Do not attempt to remove the object.
FOR *CHEMICAL BURNS TO THE EYE see p.64.*

1 Lay your child down and cradle his head in your lap to keep it still. Tell him to try not to move his eyes.

COVER injured eye with an eyepad

2 Reassure your child and then cover the injured eye with an eyepad or sterile dressing. Bandage the pad firmly, but gently, in place.

BANDAGE pad in place

3 Bandage both eyes, since movement of the good eye will cause movement of the bad eye.

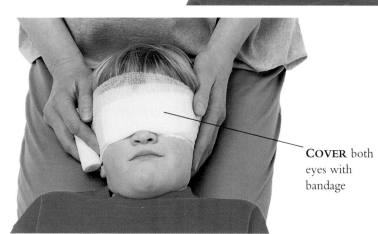

COVER both eyes with bandage

☎ CALL AN AMBULANCE OR
✚ TAKE YOUR CHILD
TO HOSPITAL
Keep him lying on his back.

52

NOSEBLEED

TILT her head forward

PINCH her nostrils together for ten minutes

1 Sit your child down with her head well forward. Ask her to breathe through her mouth, then pinch the fleshy part of her nose for ten minutes.

> **IF** *there is a watery discharge from the nose following a* HEAD INJURY *(see p. 71),*
> ✚ TAKE YOUR CHILD TO HOSPITAL

KEEP her head forward

PINCH for further ten minutes if bleeding has not stopped. Repeat if necessary

LET her dribble or spit into a bowl

2 Tell your child to spit out any excess fluid in her mouth. If the bleeding has not stopped, pinch again for ten minutes then release pressure. If the nose is still bleeding, pinch again.

53

> **IF** *the nosebleed goes on for more than 30 minutes,*
> ✚ TAKE YOUR CHILD TO HOSPITAL

CLEAN gently with cotton wool

3 Once the bleeding has stopped, use some cotton wool dipped in lukewarm water to clean around your child's nose and mouth. Advise her to rest. If your child picks at, or blows, her nose within the next few hours, the bleeding may start again.

TELL her not to blow her nose

EAR

Bleeding from inside the ear

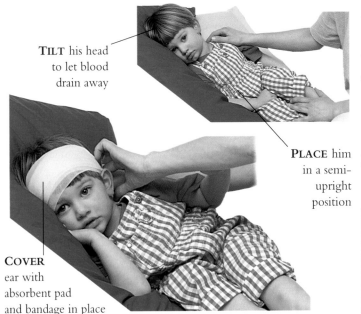

TILT his head to let blood drain away

PLACE him in a semi-upright position

COVER ear with absorbent pad and bandage in place

1 Help your child into a semi-upright position, with his head tilted towards the injured side, to allow blood to drain away.

2 Put an absorbent pad over the ear and bandage it lightly in place. Do not plug the ear.

☏ CALL A DOCTOR

> **IF** *the bleeding follows a* HEAD INJURY *(see p.71) and the fluid draining from the ear is thin and watery,*
> ☎ CALL AN AMBULANCE

54

External bleeding

PRESS on wound over a clean pad for ten minutes

1 Gently pinch the wound with a piece of gauze, pressing for ten minutes.

2 Cover her ear with a sterile dressing and lightly bandage it in place.

☏ CALL A DOCTOR

BANDAGE to keep wound covered

> **IF** *the injury is caused by an earring being ripped out, your child may need stitches.*
> ✚ TAKE YOUR CHILD TO HOSPITAL

MOUTH INJURY

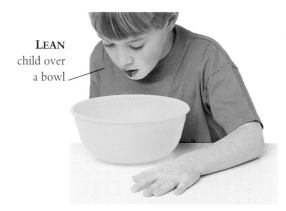

LEAN child over a bowl

DO NOT *wash out his mouth as this may disturb a blood clot.*

PRESS on wound over a clean pad for ten minutes

1 Sit your child down, with his head over a bowl into which he can dribble the blood.

2 Place a pad over the wound and pinch it between your thumb and forefinger, maintaining the pressure for ten minutes.

Knocked out tooth

HOLD a pad over the tooth socket

AN "ADULT" TOOTH *may be re-planted. Do not clean it. Put the tooth in milk.*
✚ TAKE YOUR CHILD TO THE DENTIST

1 Place a pad over the tooth socket, making sure that it is higher than the adjacent teeth so that your child can bite on it.

2 Ask your child to sit down with her hand supporting her jaw. Tell her to bite hard on the pad. A younger child may need you to hold the pad in place.

MILK TEETH *are not re-planted, but try to find the tooth to ensure that it has not been inhaled or swallowed. A dentist should check the gum.*

AMPUTATION

PRESS over a clean pad to control bleeding

RAISE the injured part

BANDAGE the pad

1 Control the blood loss by pressing firmly on the injury over a sterile dressing or clean pad. Raise the injured part above the level of your child's heart.

> **DO NOT** *use a tourniquet.*

2 Bandage or tape the dressing firmly in place. You can cover a finger with a gauze finger bandage.

☎ CALL AN AMBULANCE and tell the control it is an amputation.

> **YOU** *may need to treat your child for* SHOCK, *see p.30, and* BLEEDING, *p.46.*

Care of the amputated part

IT *is sometimes possible to "re-plant" an amputated part using microsurgery. The sooner both the child and the severed part reach hospital, the better.* **NEVER** *wash the severed part or allow it to come into direct contact with the ice.* **DO NOT** *apply cotton wool to any raw surface.*

1 Wrap the severed part in kitchen film or a plastic bag.

2 Wrap the bag in a soft fabric, such as a cotton handkerchief or gauze.

3 Put a plastic bag filled with ice cubes around the fabric. This helps preserve the severed part.

4 Put the whole package in another bag or container. Mark with the time of injury and the child's name. Give it to the ambulance attendant.

INTERNAL BLEEDING

Suspect this when signs of shock develop without obvious blood loss.

Recognising internal bleeding • *Pale, cold, and sweaty skin tinged with grey* • *A rapid pulse becoming weaker* • *Shallow, fast breathing* • *Restlessness, yawning, and sighing* • *Thirst* • *Possible loss of consciousness.*

After violent injury, there may be: • *"Pattern bruising" at the site of injury with marks from clothes or crushing objects* • *Bleeding from orifices – note what it looks like and try to take a sample to hospital.*

See HEAD INJURY *(p.71),* SHOCK *(p.30).*

☎ CALL AN AMBULANCE

> **IF** *your child loses consciousness, assess his condition (see* UNCONSCIOUS BABY *p.16;* CHILD *p.22). Be prepared to resuscitate. If breathing, place him in the* RECOVERY POSITION.

RAISE and support her legs

Lay her down with her legs raised. Check her breathing and pulse.

LOOSEN clothing

CHECK her breathing and pulse

LAY her down on a rug

COVER her with a blanket

57

CRUSH INJURY

☎ CALL AN AMBULANCE

REMOVE the object quickly

PRESS on wound to control any bleeding

> **IF** *the child has been crushed for more than ten minutes, do not remove the object, as this increases the risk of shock and further internal injury. Reassure your child.*

1 If the accident has just happened, remove the heavy object quickly.

2 Control any bleeding by pressing firmly on the wound, with your hand or a clean pad.

> **IF** *you suspect broken bones, support the injury with padding, but do not move your child until help arrives. Watch for signs of* SHOCK *(see above and p.30).*

CHEST WOUND

SUPPORT him in semi-upright position

COVER wound with your hand

PLACE clean pad over wound

COVER pad with kitchen film and secure with strapping

REASSURE him

TURN child, to lean on injured side

A chest wound may cause severe internal damage. The lungs are particularly vulnerable, and breathing problems, shock, and collapsed lungs may follow an injury. It is important to make an airtight seal over the wound to prevent air entering the cavity.

1 Cover the wound with the palm of your hand and support your child in a semi-upright position.

2 With your child supported, cover the wound with a sterile dressing or clean pad and tape it in place.

3 Create an airtight seal by covering the pad with a piece of kitchen film, secured in place with adhesive strapping.

4 Incline your child towards his injured side, supported on cushions.

IF *your child loses consciousness, assess his condition (see UNCONSCIOUS BABY p.16; CHILD p.22). Be prepared to resuscitate. If breathing, place him in the RECOVERY POSITION lying on his injured side. Check for signs of SHOCK (see p.30).*

☎ CALL AN AMBULANCE

58

ABDOMINAL WOUND

1 Lay your child down and place a cushion or pillow under her knees to ease the strain on her abdomen. Loosen any tight clothing.

BEND her knees and support her with a cushion

LAY child down gently

COVER wound with dressing

2 Reassure your child while you place a large sterile dressing over the wound. Press over the wound if your child is about to cough or vomit.

> **IF** *part of the intestine is showing, cover it with a polythene bag or kitchen film before dressing the wound.*

TAPE dressing in place

3 Use adhesive tape to secure the dressing lightly in place. Continue to reassure her and watch for any change in her condition; look particularly for signs of SHOCK (p.30).
☎ CALL AN AMBULANCE

> **IF** *your child loses consciousness, assess her condition (see UNCONSCIOUS BABY p.16; CHILD p.22). Be prepared to resuscitate.*

59

BURNS AND SCALDS

For information on dealing with fires, see ACTION IN AN EMERGENCY p.11.

DO NOT *remove any clothing or material that may be sticking to the burned area as this may cause further damage to the skin.*

COOL burn with cold water for at least ten minutes

IF *no cold water is available, use another cool liquid such as milk.*

✚ TAKE YOUR CHILD TO HOSPITAL
OR ☎ CALL AN AMBULANCE

1 To stop the burning process and relieve pain, cool the burn with cold water for at least ten minutes.

DO NOT *immerse young children in cold water as this can cause hypothermia.*

REMOVE cooled clothing and cool injury again

2 Once cooled, remove clothing from the burned area and, if the pain persists, cool again. Cut around any material sticking to the skin. Remove restrictive clothing from the area of a burn before it begins to swell.

DO NOT *touch the burn or burst any blisters.*

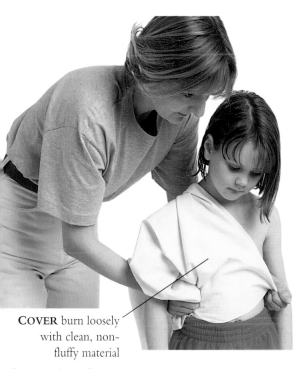

3 Cover the burn with clean, non-fluffy material to protect it from infection. You can use a clean sheet or pillow case. The dressing does not need to be secured. Do not apply lotions, fat, or ointment.

COVER burn loosely with clean, non-fluffy material

> **DO NOT** *give her anything to eat or drink and watch for signs of SHOCK (see p.30).*

> **IF** *she loses consciousness, assess her condition (see UNCONSCIOUS BABY p.16; child p.22). Be prepared to resuscitate. If breathing, place her in the RECOVERY POSITION.*

Alternative dressings To dress a burned hand or foot you can use a plastic bag or clean kitchen film. Secure this with a bandage or plaster around the bag, not the skin.

PROTECT with clean plastic bag

PROTECT with kitchen film

61

Burns to the mouth and throat

Burns in this area are very dangerous as they cause swelling and inflammation of the air passages, giving a serious risk of suffocation. Act quickly. If necessary, loosen clothing from around his neck. Give him cold water to sip.

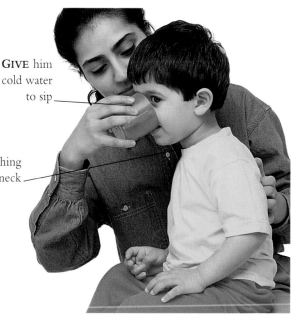

GIVE him cold water to sip

LOOSEN clothing around his neck

☎ CALL AN AMBULANCE

> **IF** *your child develops breathing difficulties, assess his condition (see UNCONSCIOUS BABY p.16; CHILD p.22). Be prepared to resuscitate.*

ELECTRICAL BURN

An electric shock from a low-voltage source can result in burns. These may occur at both the point of entry and the point of exit of an electrical current. See ELECTRICAL INJURY (p.12), SHOCK (p.30).

DO NOT *approach your child directly until you are sure the electrical current is switched off.*

IF *your child loses consciousness, assess her condition (see UNCONSCIOUS BABY p.16; child p.22). Be prepared to resuscitate. If breathing, place her in the RECOVERY POSITION.*

COOL burns with cold water for at least ten minutes

1 Hold the injured area under cold, running water for at least ten minutes to cool the burn.

2 Protect the burn by covering it with clean, non-fluffy material or with a plastic bag, held or taped in place.

+ TAKE YOUR CHILD TO HOSPITAL

COVER with a clean plastic bag

62

CHEMICAL BURN TO SKIN

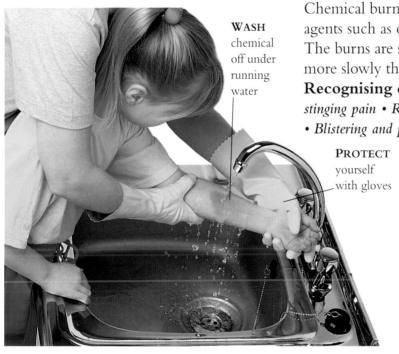

WASH chemical off under running water

Chemical burns can be caused by household agents such as oven cleaner or paint stripper. The burns are serious but signs develop more slowly than for thermal burns.
Recognising chemical burns • *Fierce, stinging pain* • *Redness or staining,* followed by • *Blistering and peeling*

PROTECT yourself with gloves

1 Wash away all traces of the chemical by holding the affected area under plenty of running water.

NOTE *the name of the substance that caused the burn. Wear protective rubber gloves, and beware of fumes. See FUME INHALATION p.43, and SWALLOWED CHEMICALS p.65.*

63

Removing clothes

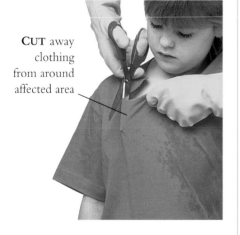

CUT away clothing from around affected area

Cut off clothing from the affected area, unless you can slip it off without touching other parts of the body. Avoid cutting through the affected area – cut around it instead.

COVER burn loosely with clean, non-fluffy material

2 Loosely cover the burn with clean, non-fluffy material, such as a pillow case. This avoids constriction when the wound swells. You can wet the pillow case to cool and soothe the burn.

✚ TAKE YOUR CHILD TO HOSPITAL

CHEMICAL BURNS TO EYE

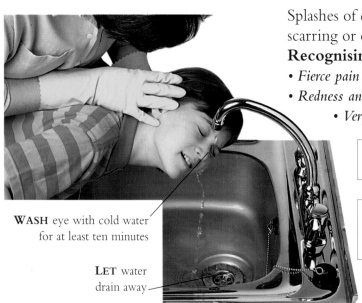

Splashes of chemicals in the eye can cause scarring or even blindness.

Recognising chemical burns to the eye
- *Fierce pain in the eye* • *Difficulty opening the eye*
- *Redness and swelling in and around the eye*
  - *Very watery eye*

WASH eye with cold water for at least ten minutes

LET water drain away

> **DO NOT** *let your child rub her eye.*

> **THE EYE** *will be shut in spasm and pain, so gently pull the eyelids open.*

USE a jug, if this is easier

BE careful not to splash water in her face

1 Hold your child over a basin, with the good eye uppermost, and gently run cold water over the contaminated eye for at least ten minutes. Wear protective gloves. Make sure that both sides of the eyelid are thoroughly washed and that the water drains away from her face. You may find it easier to use a jug. Avoid splashing the good eye with contaminated water.

COVER eye with clean pad and bandage in place

2 When the injured eye is thoroughly washed, cover it with a sterile eye pad or dressing. Bandage the pad in place and secure this with tape.

✚ TAKE YOUR CHILD TO HOSPITAL

64

SWALLOWED CHEMICALS

WASH your child's lips and mouth gently

IF *you think your child has swallowed anything poisonous,* ☎ CALL A DOCTOR

1 Wipe away any residual chemical around the mouth and face.

2 Her lips may be burned or discoloured, so give her frequent sips of cold water or milk.

HELP her take sips of cold water or milk

DO NOT *try to make your child vomit as this can cause further harm.*

65

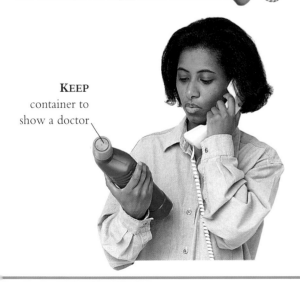

KEEP container to show a doctor

3 Find out what chemical your child swallowed and telephone a doctor with the information. This will help determine the correct medical treatment.

IF *your child loses consciousness, assess her condition (see* UNCONSCIOUS BABY, *p.16;* CHILD *p.22). Be prepared to resuscitate. If breathing, place her in the* RECOVERY POSITION.

DRUG POISONING

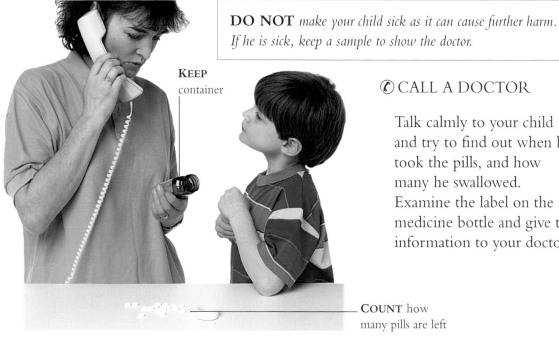

> **DO NOT** *make your child sick as it can cause further harm. If he is sick, keep a sample to show the doctor.*

KEEP container

☏ CALL A DOCTOR

Talk calmly to your child and try to find out when he took the pills, and how many he swallowed. Examine the label on the medicine bottle and give the information to your doctor.

COUNT how many pills are left

If the child is unconscious

☏ CALL AN AMBULANCE

CLEAR his mouth, if necessary

1 Open his mouth. Hook out with a finger any drugs that you can see.

> **TRY** *to find out what drugs he has taken and how much he has swallowed.*

OPEN airway   **CHECK** for breathing   **CHECK** his pulse

2 Open his airway. Check his breathing and pulse (see UNCONSCIOUS BABY p.16; CHILD p.22). Be prepared to resuscitate. If he is breathing, place him in the RECOVERY POSITION. Stay with him until help arrives.

PLACE him in recovery position if breathing

ALCOHOL POISONING

EVEN *a small amount of alcohol may harm a young child.*

Recognising alcohol poisoning
• *A strong smell of alcohol* • *Flushed and moist face* • *Slurred speech* • *Staggering* • *Deep noisy breathing* • *Nausea* • *Bounding pulse*

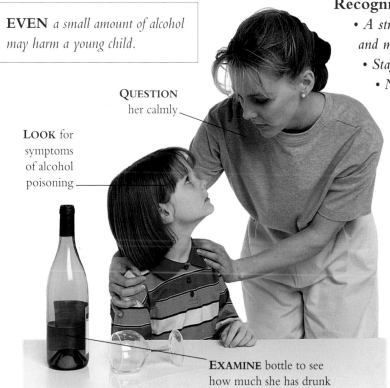

QUESTION her calmly

LOOK for symptoms of alcohol poisoning

EXAMINE bottle to see how much she has drunk

✆ CALL A DOCTOR

Allow your child to rest where you can watch over her. Place a bowl nearby in case she is sick. If she falls asleep, check her to make sure she can be easily roused. If she is very drowsy, or seems unconscious, see below.

67

If the child is unconscious

☎ CALL AN AMBULANCE

CHECK for breathing

CHECK her pulse

OPEN airway

PLACE her in recovery position if breathing

KEEP *your child warm. Alcohol dilates the blood vessels, which can cause hypothermia.*

Open her airway. Check her breathing and pulse (see UNCONSCIOUS BABY p.16; CHILD p.22). Be prepared to resuscitate. If she is breathing, place her in the RECOVERY POSITION. Stay with her until help arrives.

PLANT POISONING

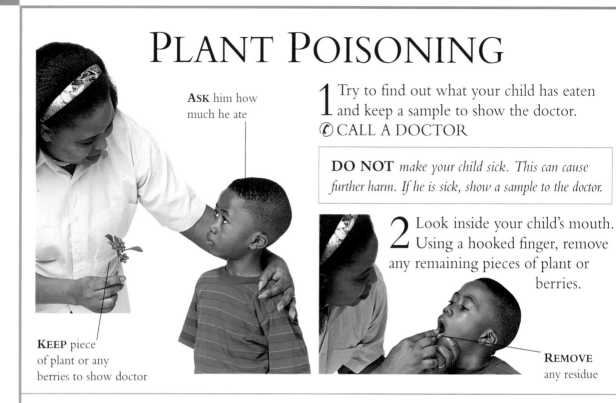

ASK him how much he ate

KEEP piece of plant or any berries to show doctor

1 Try to find out what your child has eaten and keep a sample to show the doctor.
☏ CALL A DOCTOR

> **DO NOT** *make your child sick. This can cause further harm. If he is sick, show a sample to the doctor.*

2 Look inside your child's mouth. Using a hooked finger, remove any remaining pieces of plant or berries.

REMOVE any residue

If the child is unconscious

CLEAR his mouth, if necessary

1 Open his mouth. Hook out with a finger any pieces of plant that you can see.

☎ CALL AN AMBULANCE

2 Open his airway. Check his breathing and pulse (see UNCONSCIOUS BABY p.16; CHILD p.22). Be prepared to resuscitate. If he is breathing, place him in the RECOVERY POSITION. Stay with him until the ambulance arrives.

OPEN airway

CHECK for breathing

CHECK his pulse

PLACE him in recovery position if breathing

SCALP WOUND

PLACE a clean pad onto wound

APPLY firm, steady pressure

1 Cover the injury with a clean pad or sterile dressing that is larger than the wound. Scalp wounds can bleed dramatically, so press firmly on the pad and the wound to control the bleeding. Place another pad on top, if necessary. Keep pressing.

BANDAGE pad in place

SECURE bandage firmly but not too tightly

2 Bandage the dressing firmly in place. If the bleeding continues, apply pressure again with your hand.

IF *the wound has been caused by a blow to the head,*
☏ CALL A DOCTOR
(see also CONCUSSION p. 70; SKULL FRACTURE p. 71).

69

LAY your child down

KEEP her head and shoulders slightly raised

3 Help your child to lie down with her head and shoulders slightly raised. Watch for any changes.

IF *she deteriorates or loses consciousness, assess her condition (see UNCONSCIOUS BABY p. 16; CHILD p. 22). Be prepared to resuscitate. If breathing, place her in the RECOVERY POSITION.*
☎ CALL AN AMBULANCE

CONCUSSION

The brain may be "shaken" by a violent blow causing concussion. The period of unconsciousness is brief and followed by complete recovery. You should be able to distinguish between a bump on the head with no concussion, a brief period of concussion (less than 20 seconds), and an extended period of unconsciousness.

Recognising concussion • *Brief loss of consciousness, dizziness or nausea on recovery*
• *Loss of memory of immediately preceding events*
• *A mild headache*

Conscious child

TREAT any wound or bump

WATCH for abnormal behaviour

If your child has bumped his head, sit him down and treat any minor bruise or wound with a cold compress.

> **WATCH** *for signs of abnormal behaviour. If he does not recover fully within a few minutes,* ℂ CALL A DOCTOR.

Child who regains consciousness quickly

1 If your child has been "knocked out", even briefly,
ℂ CALL A DOCTOR

2 Make her rest and watch her closely. If she does not recover completely within 30 minutes,
☎ CALL AN AMBULANCE

WATCH child carefully for abnormal behaviour

MAKE sure she rests

Unconscious child

OPEN airway

CHECK his pulse

CHECK for breathing

PLACE him in the recovery position if breathing

☎ CALL AN AMBULANCE

Open his airway. Check his breathing and pulse (see UNCONSCIOUS BABY p.16; CHILD p.22). If breathing, place him in the RECOVERY POSITION. Stay with him until the ambulance arrives.

SKULL FRACTURE

Fractures of the skull are potentially very serious injuries and require urgent medical attention to minimise the risk of damage to the brain and the possibility of infection.
Recognising a skull fracture • *A wound or bruise on the head* • *A soft area on the scalp* • *Impaired consciousness* • *Deterioration in level* of response • *Clear fluid from the nose or ear* • *Blood showing in the white of the eye* • *Distortion of the head or face.*

☎ CALL AN AMBULANCE

> **IF** *you suspect BACK OR NECK INJURIES, see pp. 73-74.*

Unconscious child

OPEN airway

CHECK for breathing

CHECK her pulse

PLACE her in recovery position if breathing

1 Open her airway. Check her breathing and pulse (see UNCONSCIOUS BABY, p.16; CHILD, p.22).

2 If she is breathing, place her in the RECOVERY POSITION. Stay with her and watch for any change in her condition while waiting for the ambulance to arrive.

71

Delayed reaction

There may be a serious reaction to a head injury hours or even days later. Cerebral compression is a condition caused by blood accumulating within the skull and putting pressure on the brain following a head injury.
Recognising cerebral compression
• *Disorientation and confusion* • *A severe headache* • *Impaired consciousness* • *Noisy breathing, becoming slow* • *A slow but strong pulse* • *Unequal pupils* • *Weakness or paralysis* • *A raised temperature*
Be prepared to resuscitate (see UNCONSCIOUS BABY p.16; CHILD, p.22).

☎ CALL AN AMBULANCE

BROKEN NOSE/CHEEKBONE

APPLY cold compress to injury

1 Sit your child down and apply a cold compress to the injured part. This helps to reduce the swelling. Hold the compress in place for about 30 minutes.

2 If your child's nose is bleeding heavily, ask her to sit with her head over a bowl and to pinch her nostrils together.

PINCH nostrils together to stop bleeding

SIT your child well forward over bowl

IF *pinching her nose hurts too much, simply ask her to sit forward and give her a soft pad or towel to soak up the blood.*

✚TAKE YOUR CHILD TO HOSPITAL

BROKEN JAW

Recognising a broken jaw
• *Tender, swollen, bruised jaw* • *Teeth may be out of line*

HELP her to lean forward

1 Sit her down with her head well forward. Tell her not to swallow, but to let any blood or saliva drain away.

HOLD pad against jaw and support jaw with your hand

IF *she loses consciousness, assess her condition (see* UNCONSCIOUS BABY, p.16; CHILD p.22). *Be prepared to resuscitate. If breathing, place her in the* RECOVERY POSITION.

☎ CALL AN AMBULANCE

2 Make a soft pad and hold it firmly under her injured jaw. Do not bandage the pad in place in case she is sick. Continue to support the jaw on the journey to the hospital.

✚ TAKE YOUR CHILD TO HOSPITAL

BACK AND NECK INJURIES
The conscious child

☎ CALL AN AMBULANCE

> **DO NOT** *move the injured child unless his life is in danger.* **IF** *you do have to move him, try to do so in "one piece", taking care not to twist or bend the neck or spine.*

REASSURE your child

HOLD his head in your hands

KEEP his back straight

1 Reassure your child and tell him not to move. Steady and support his head and neck by placing your hands over his ears and keeping his head in line with his spine. Be careful not to pull on his neck.

MAINTAIN support of his head

2 Keep his head supported in this position until help arrives. Ask someone to put rolled blankets or towels around his neck and shoulders for extra support.

PLACE rolled blankets around his head and shoulders

CONTINUE to support his head

3 Get a helper to arrange rolled towels or blankets around your child's neck and shoulders and either side of his body while you continue to keep his head steady.

PLACE folded blankets or towels either side of his body

73

BACK AND NECK INJURIES
The unconscious child

☎ CALL AN AMBULANCE

1 Keep your child's head, trunk, and toes in a straight line.

KEEP head and body aligned

> **MOVE** *your child only if you think his life is in immediate danger.*

OPEN airway

LIFT his chin

2 Place two fingers under the chin and lift the jaw very gently to open the airway. At the same time, place your hand on his forehead and tilt his head back slightly.

TILT head very gently and support it

3 Check for breathing (see UNCONSCIOUS BABY p.16; CHILD p.22).

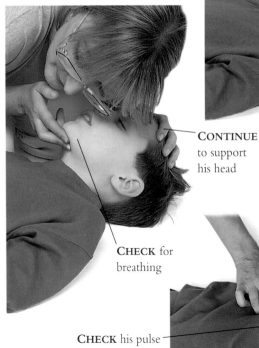

CONTINUE to support his head

CHECK for breathing

CHECK his pulse

4 With the palm of your hand still supporting your child's head, check his pulse (see UNCONSCIOUS BABY p.16; CHILD p.22). Be prepared to resuscitate.

CONTINUE to support his head

74

Modified recovery position

GET help to support head and neck

STRAIGHTEN his leg very gently

DRAW furthest arm across his chest

BRING nearest arm out, elbow bent, palm uppermost

LIFT and bend the leg furthest away from you

KEEP head supported and in line with his trunk

KEEP head and neck supported

EASE child over, keeping his head aligned

DRAW over his knee

BEND uppermost leg to prevent him rolling forward

If the ambulance has not yet arrived, place your child in a modified recovery position that keeps the head and trunk aligned at all times.

1 Ask a helper to support your child's head with her hands. Grasp the thigh of the leg furthest from you. Gently lift and bend the leg. Draw the arm furthest from you across the child's chest.

2 Draw over his knee and ease him round gently. Keep his head and trunk aligned.

3 With your child turned onto his side and his head tilted back, support him in this position until help arrives. Monitor his breathing and pulse. Be prepared to resuscitate, see below and UNCONSCIOUS BABY p.16; CHILD p.22.

75

Rolling an unconscious child

KEEP head in line with body while he is turned

ONE helper supports arms and legs and pulls gently

ONE helper keeps trunk straight

If you need to resuscitate a child who has stopped breathing, use the "log-roll" technique to turn him onto his back. It is vital to keep the child's head, trunk and feet in a straight line. You will need helpers to do this safely. While one adult holds the child's head, two others should gently straighten the limbs and roll the child over in one synchronised movement. You can then resuscitate (see UNCONSCIOUS BABY p.16; CHILD p.22).

BROKEN LEG

SUPPORT leg at joints above and below injury

1 Lay your child down gently and support his leg at the ankle and knee joints. Ask someone to help you, if possible.

2 Steady the injured leg with padding. Place one rolled-up blanket outside the injured limb and one between the legs. If necessary, cover him with another blanket to keep him warm.

MAKE a J-shaped pad with a rolled blanket and place it around his leg

☎ CALL AN AMBULANCE

Making broad-fold and narrow-fold bandages

TAKE a triangular bandage

BROAD-FOLD BANDAGE

FOLD bandage in half to make a broad-fold

FOLD top point over to touch the base

NARROW-FOLD BANDAGE

FOLD bandage in half again to make a narrow-fold bandage

Tying a reef knot

CROSS the left end (yellow) over the right (blue)

TAKE the yellow under and through

PASS the yellow over the blue and through the gap

PULL the ends firmly

How to splint an injured leg

PLACE plenty of soft padding between the legs

SUPPORT injured leg

TIE narrow-fold bandage in figure-of-eight at ankles and feet

SLIDE broad-fold under knee and tie ends together

TIE reef knots on uninjured side

TIE broad-fold bandages at knees and above injury

1 If the ambulance will be longer than 20 minutes, splint the injured leg. Gently pad between the thighs, knees and ankles using rolled up towels or small blankets. Carefully bring the uninjured leg alongside the broken limb.

2 Tie a narrow-fold figure-of-eight bandage around the feet and ankles to immobilise the leg.

3 Tie broad-fold bandages around the knee and above the injury.

BROKEN PELVIS

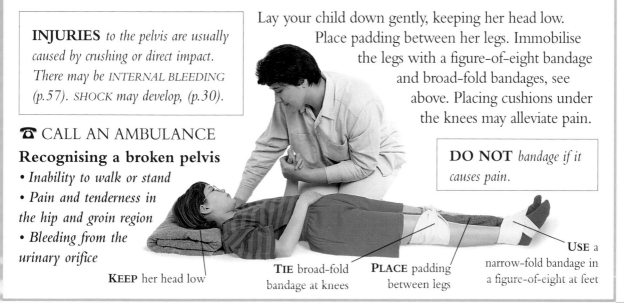

INJURIES *to the pelvis are usually caused by crushing or direct impact. There may be INTERNAL BLEEDING (p.57). SHOCK may develop, (p.30).*

☎ CALL AN AMBULANCE

Recognising a broken pelvis
- *Inability to walk or stand*
- *Pain and tenderness in the hip and groin region*
- *Bleeding from the urinary orifice*

Lay your child down gently, keeping her head low. Place padding between her legs. Immobilise the legs with a figure-of-eight bandage and broad-fold bandages, see above. Placing cushions under the knees may alleviate pain.

DO NOT *bandage if it causes pain.*

KEEP her head low

TIE broad-fold bandage at knees

PLACE padding between legs

USE a narrow-fold bandage in a figure-of-eight at feet

KNEE INJURY

1 Help your child to lie down, then slide a pillow under the injured knee to provide support. Pad around the injured knee with cotton wool or a soft dressing.

2 Use a roller bandage to keep the padding in place, working from the child's injured side.

SUPPORT his knee with a pillow

WRAP padding around joint and bandage

KEEP him comfortable

> **DO NOT** *attempt to force the knee straight as this may cause further injury.*

> **DO NOT** *allow the child to eat, drink, or walk.*

✚ TAKE YOUR CHILD TO HOSPITAL
OR ☎ CALL AN AMBULANCE

78

BROKEN FOOT

Fractures of the foot are usually caused by crushing.
Recognising a broken foot
• *Bruising and swelling* • *Stiffness*
• *Difficulty in walking*

Sit your child down. Raise and support the injured foot. Hold an icepack against the injury. Bandage it in place to relieve pain.

✚ TAKE YOUR CHILD TO HOSPITAL

REDUCE swelling with an ice pack

KEEP leg elevated

BROKEN COLLAR BONE

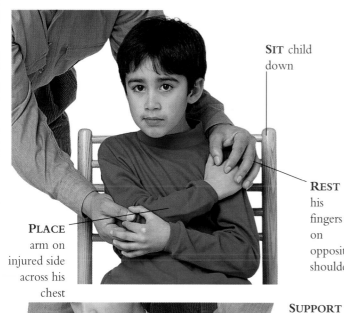

SIT child down

REST his fingers on opposite shoulder

PLACE arm on injured side across his chest

The collar bone may be broken by indirect force, if a child falls onto his outstretched hand, or by a blow to his shoulder.

Recognising a broken collar bone • *Pain and tenderness increased by movement* • *Head turned and inclined to the injured side*

1 Sit your child down and gently bring the arm on the injured side across his chest. Ask him to support his elbow in his hand.

SUPPORT arm in an elevation sling

PLACE padding between arm and body

2 Place your child's arm in an ELEVATION SLING for support (see p.111). Use REEF KNOTS (see p.76).

3 Secure the arm with a BROAD-FOLD BANDAGE (see p.76 and below).

✚ TAKE YOUR CHILD TO HOSPITAL

TIE a broad-fold bandage around arm and body

79

Tying a broad-fold bandage around a sling

SLIDE padding between arm and body

PLACE a broad-fold bandage around body and arm

SECURE with a reef knot tied on uninjured side

A sling will support an injured arm, but a broad-fold bandage provides extra support if you need to take your child on a journey.

BROKEN ARM

PLACE arm across chest

ASK him to support injury

PLACE padding around injury

SUPPORT arm in a sling

TIE a broad-fold bandage around arm and chest

The treatment described below is suitable for injuries to the upper arm, forearm, and wrist.

1 Sit your child down and if possible get him to support his injured arm in his hand.

2 Place a pad between his arm and his chest to immobilise and cushion the injured limb.

3 Put the injured limb in an ARM SLING (see p.110), secured with a REEF KNOT (see p.76).

4 For additional support, place a BROAD-FOLD BANDAGE over the sling and around your child's arm and chest (see p.76 and 79).

✚ TAKE YOUR CHILD TO HOSPITAL

80

BROKEN ELBOW

LAY child down

PLACE injured arm across his body

PUT soft padding between his arm and body

BANDAGE upper arm to chest with broad-fold bandage

Elbow injuries need special care and early treatment in hospital.

Recognising a broken elbow • *Pain increased by attempted movement* • *Stiffness* • *Swelling or bruising*

DO NOT *attempt to straighten or bend the elbow. Make sure the bandages are not too tight.*

☎ CALL AN AMBULANCE

SECURE wrist and lower arm to hips with broad-fold bandage

BROKEN RIBS

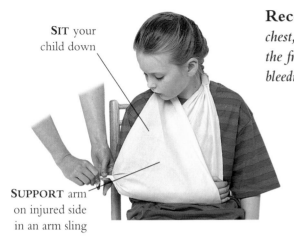

SIT your child down

SUPPORT arm on injured side in an arm sling

Recognising broken ribs • *Child has had a blow to chest, a heavy fall, or has been crushed* • *Sharp pain at the fracture site* • *Pain on breathing* • *Signs of internal bleeding* • *Open wound over the fracture site*

Support the arm on the injured side in an ARM SLING (see p.110).

✚ TAKE YOUR CHILD TO HOSPITAL

> **IF** *the child has a CHEST WOUND (see p.58) or INTERNAL BLEEDING (see p.57),*
>
> ☎ CALL AN AMBULANCE

Open or multiple rib fractures

LEAN child towards injured side in semi-upright position

SEAL wound with pad and kitchen wrap taped in place

RAISE arm on injured side across his chest

PUT arm on injured side in elevation sling

☎ CALL AN AMBULANCE

Treat any open wound and support the chest wall to safeguard breathing (see also CHEST WOUND p.58).

1 Help the child into a semi-upright position supported by pillows. Incline his body towards the injured side. Cover any wounds to the chest wall using a sterile pad sealed with kitchen film.

2 Place the arm on the injured side across your child's chest.

3 Support the raised arm in an ELEVATION SLING (see p.111). Keep him as comfortable as possible while you wait for the ambulance.

> **IF** *your child loses consciousness or develops breathing difficulties, assess his condition (see UNCONSCIOUS BABY, p.16; CHILD p.22). Be prepared to resuscitate.*

81

BROKEN HAND

WRAP hand in soft padding

1 Wrap the injured hand in soft cotton wool padding. Raise your child's hand, supporting it to minimise swelling.

> **IF** *there is a wound, control the bleeding by raising the hand and applying gentle pressure over a clean, non-fluffy pad.*
>
> **COVER** any wound with a non-fluffy dressing
>
> **APPLY** pressure to control bleeding

2 Place your child's arm in an ELEVATION SLING (see p.111) to reduce swelling and prevent movement of the injured hand.

SUPPORT hand and arm in elevation sling

TIE broad-fold bandage around arm and body

3 Tie a BROAD-FOLD BANDAGE (see p.76 and 79) around the arm, securing it with a knot tied on the uninjured side.

+ TAKE YOUR CHILD TO HOSPITAL

TRAPPED FINGERS

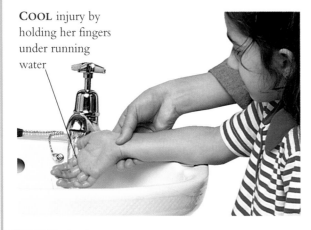

COOL injury by holding her fingers under running water

Hold the fingers under cold running water for a few minutes to relieve the pain and minimise swelling. If the fingers still hurt, apply a COLD COMPRESS (see p.84).

> **IF** *after half an hour the fingers are still swollen and movement is impaired, they may be broken.*
>
> **+** TAKE YOUR CHILD TO HOSPITAL

SPRAINED ANKLE

Suspect an ankle sprain if your child can't take her full weight on her foot after a fall or wrench.

RAISE and support foot to minimise swelling

REMOVE sock and shoe

1 Sit your child down to rest her foot. Raise her foot and gently remove her sock and shoe before swelling occurs.

APPLY a cold compress

KEEP ankle raised

2 To minimise swelling, apply a COLD COMPRESS, such as a flannel wrung out in cold water or an icepack (see overleaf).

WRAP with cotton wool padding

KEEP ankle raised and supported

BANDAGE padding firmly in place

3 Wrap the ankle with a thick layer of cotton wool. Bandage the cotton wool firmly in place. Keep the ankle raised.

ℂ CALL A DOCTOR

IF *you suspect a* BROKEN FOOT, *see p.78.*
✚ TAKE YOUR CHILD TO HOSPITAL

83

BRUISES AND SWELLINGS

After a fall or bump, bruising and swelling may develop rapidly. Resting, cooling, and elevating the injury will alleviate symptoms.

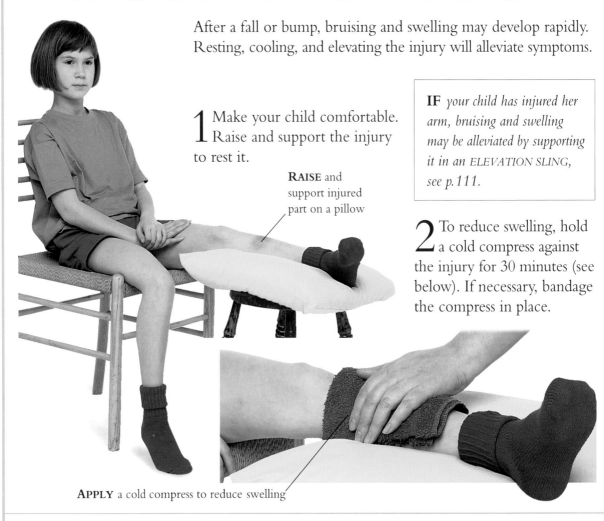

1 Make your child comfortable. Raise and support the injury to rest it.

RAISE and support injured part on a pillow

IF *your child has injured her arm, bruising and swelling may be alleviated by supporting it in an* ELEVATION SLING, *see p.111.*

2 To reduce swelling, hold a cold compress against the injury for 30 minutes (see below). If necessary, bandage the compress in place.

APPLY a cold compress to reduce swelling

Making a cold compress

A cold compress minimises swelling and pain by reducing blood flow to the injured area. Leave a compress on the injury for about 30 minutes, changing it as necessary. If possible, the compress should be left uncovered, but if you need to secure it in place, use a gauze bandage or other open-weave material.

Cloth: wring it out in cold water and replace every ten minutes.

Bag of frozen peas: wrap in a light towel before placing it on the injury.

Ice: fill a plastic bag two-thirds full of ice and add a little salt to help the ice melt, then seal.

SPLINTER

1 Clean the area around the splinter with soap and warm water.

WASH around splinter with warm water

> **IF** *your child is not inoculated against* TETANUS *(p.50),* © CALL A DOCTOR

> **DO NOT** *poke at the area with a needle.*

2 Sterilise a pair of tweezers by passing them through a flame. Leave the tweezers to cool. Don't touch the ends or wipe off the soot.

STERILISE tweezers in a flame

SUPPORT child's hand

GRASP splinter and pull straight out

85

3 Grasp the splinter as close to the skin as possible, and draw it back out at the angle it went in.

> **IF** *the splinter doesn't come out easily, or if it breaks,* © CALL A DOCTOR

SQUEEZE area to encourage a little bleeding

4 Squeeze the wound to encourage a little bleeding that will flush out dirt. Wash the area again, pat it dry thoroughly, and cover with a plaster.

EYE

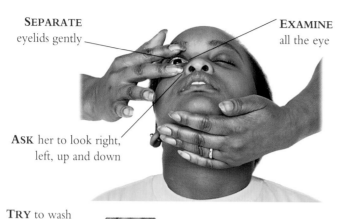

SEPARATE eyelids gently

EXAMINE all the eye

ASK her to look right, left, up and down

DO NOT *touch, or attempt to remove, any foreign body that is sticking to, or embedded in, the eye, (see below).*

1 Sit your child down, facing the light. Separate the eyelids. Ask her to look right, left, up, and down. Examine all of the eye.

TRY to wash out foreign body

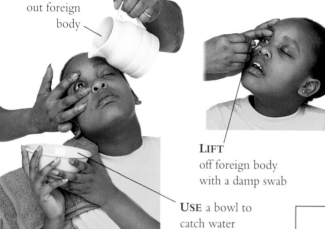

LIFT off foreign body with a damp swab

USE a bowl to catch water

2 If you can see the foreign body, wash it out using a jug of clean water. Tilt her head and aim for the inner corner so that water will wash over the eye. Or, use a damp swab or damp handkerchief to lift it off.

3 If an object is under the eyelid, you can ask an older child to clear it by lifting the upper eyelid over the lower. You will need to do this for a younger child; wrap her in a towel first to stop her grabbing your arms.

IF *eye is still red or sore,*
✚TAKE HER TO HOSPITAL

LIFT upper eyelid over lower lid

A foreign body that cannot be removed

Cover the eye with a pad and bandage so that a gentle pressure is exerted. Then bandage both eyes, to prevent movement of the good eye causing movement of the injured eye. Reassure her.

✚TAKE HER TO HOSPITAL

COVER injured eye with an eyepad

BANDAGE both eyes

86

EAR

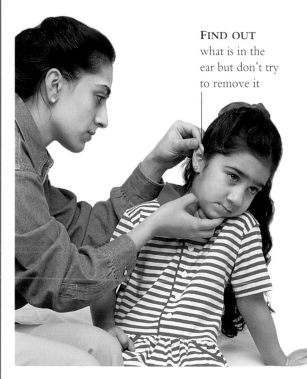

FIND OUT what is in the ear but don't try to remove it

Children often push things into their ears. A hard object may become stuck, causing pain and temporary deafness; it may damage the ear drum.

DO NOT *attempt to remove the object.*

Reassure your child and ask her what she put into her ear. Don't try to remove the object, even if you can see it.

✚ TAKE YOUR CHILD TO HOSPITAL

An insect in the ear

If an insect flies or crawls into the ear your child may be very alarmed. Sit her down and support her head with the affected ear uppermost. Gently flood the ear with tepid water so that the insect floats out.

IF *you can't remove the insect,* ✚TAKE YOUR CHILD TO HOSPITAL

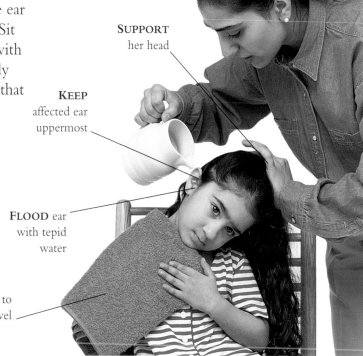

SUPPORT her head

KEEP affected ear uppermost

FLOOD ear with tepid water

ASK her to hold a towel

NOSE

Recognising foreign body in the nose

• *Difficult or noisy breathing through nose* • *Swelling of nose* • *Smelly or blood-stained discharge indicates object has been present for a while*

Calm and reassure your child and tell him to breathe through his mouth.

ASK him to breathe through his mouth

> **DO NOT** *attempt to remove the object.*
> ✚TAKE YOUR CHILD TO HOSPITAL

SWALLOWED OBJECT

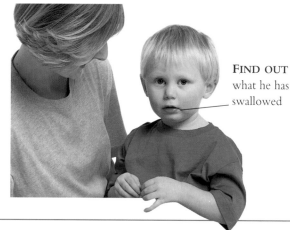

FIND OUT what he has swallowed

Find out what your child has swallowed. If the object is small and smooth like a pebble or a coin, there is little danger.

✆ CALL A DOCTOR

> **IF** *the object is sharp or large, don't give your child anything to eat or drink.*
> ✚TAKE YOUR CHILD TO HOSPITAL

INHALED FOREIGN BODY

Small, smooth objects can slip into the air passages. Peanuts are a danger in young children as they can be inhaled into the lungs.

Your child will cough violently. Put him over your knee and give sharp slaps between the shoulder blades. If he continues to choke, see CHOKING BABY p.36; CHILD p.38.

✆ CALL A DOCTOR OR
✚ TAKE HIM TO HOSPITAL

PUT him over your knee with head lower than chest

GIVE sharp slaps between shoulder blades

ANIMAL BITE
Superficial bite

WASH wound with soap and warm, running water

DRY wound and cover with a plaster

> **MAKE** *sure he is protected against tetanus infection (see p.50).*

1 Wash the wound thoroughly, using soap and warm water. Rinse the wound under running water for at least five minutes to wash away any dirt.

2 Gently, but thoroughly, pat the wound dry with a clean pad or tissue. Cover it with a plaster or a small sterile dressing.

✆ CALL A DOCTOR

Serious bite

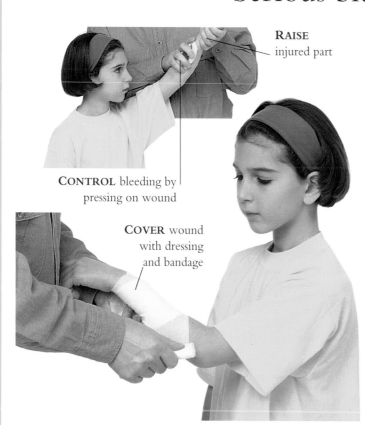

RAISE injured part

CONTROL bleeding by pressing on wound

COVER wound with dressing and bandage

1 Apply direct pressure over the wound, preferably over a clean dressing or pad. Lift and support the injured part above the level of your child's heart.

> **IF** *the bleeding is severe, see* BLEEDING, *p.46.*

2 Cover the wound with a sterile dressing or pad and bandage firmly in place.
✚ TAKE YOUR CHILD TO HOSPITAL

> **IF** *your child is bitten by an animal while you are abroad, or if the bite comes from an animal smuggled into the UK, you must take your child to hospital for anti-rabies injections.*

INSECT STING

KEEP injured part still

HOLD sting at base

PULL out sting carefully

1 If the sting is still in the skin, remove it with tweezers. Grasp the sting as close to the skin as possible and carefully pull it out. Don't grasp the sting at the top. You may squeeze the poison sac and the poison will enter the wound.

IF *your child collapses, she may be allergic to the sting. Follow the treatment for* ANAPHYLACTIC SHOCK, *opposite.*

Sting in mouth

To reduce swelling, give your child an ice cube to suck or cold water to drink.

�ℭ CALL A DOCTOR

IF her breathing becomes difficult, ☎ CALL AN AMBULANCE

PLACE a cold compress over injury

2 Cool the area with a COLD COMPRESS (see p.84) to minimise the pain and swelling. Leave the compress in place until the pain is relieved, about ten minutes. Rest the injured part.

NETTLE RASH

To relieve the itching, dab the rash with cotton wool soaked in calamine lotion. Alternatively, place a COLD COMPRESS (see p.84) over the rash until the pain is relieved, about ten minutes. If the rash is extensive, *ℭ* CALL A DOCTOR.

SOOTHE rash by dabbing with calamine lotion

ANAPHYLACTIC SHOCK

This is a severe allergic reaction that may develop within a few minutes following the injection of a particular drug, the sting of an insect or marine creature, or the ingestion of a particular food.

The reaction causes constriction of the air passages. Swelling of the face and neck increases the risk of suffocation.

Recognising anaphylactic shock
- *Anxiety* • *Red, blotchy skin* • *Swelling of the face and neck* • *Puffiness around the eyes*
- *Wheezing* • *Difficult breathing* • *Rapid pulse*

☎ CALL AN AMBULANCE

> **IF** *your child loses consciousness, assess his condition (see* UNCONSCIOUS BABY *p.16;* CHILD *p.22). If breathing, place him in the* RECOVERY POSITION. *Be prepared to resuscitate.*

> **A CHILD** *with a known allergy may have medication to take in case of an attack. Use this medication as soon as the attack starts. Follow the directions carefully.*

Help your child into the position which most relieves his breathing difficulty. Talk to him calmly and reassure him while you wait for the ambulance to arrive.

SUPPORT him in a position that helps his breathing

LOOSEN tight clothing at neck and waist

91

MARINE STINGS

Jellyfish sting

Jellyfish venom is contained in stinging cells that stick to a child's skin. The sting is painful, but not usually serious. A similar reaction is produced by sea anemones and corals.

APPLY a paste of baking soda and water

OR

DUST talcum powder over affected area

> **IF** *your child develops a severe allergic reaction, see* ANAPHYLACTIC SHOCK *p.91.* ☎ CALL AN AMBULANCE

Make a paste of baking soda and water and apply it to the wound.

OR

Dust a dry powder, such as talcum powder or meat tenderiser, over the skin around the injury.

> **IF** *the skin is very red and painful,*
> ✚TAKE YOUR CHILD TO HOSPITAL

92

Weever fish sting

When trodden on, the spines from weever fish can puncture the skin, causing painful swelling and soreness. The spines may break off and become embedded in the foot.

Immerse the injury in water as hot as your child can bear for at least 30 minutes. Top up as the water cools but be careful not to scald her.

> **IF** *any spines remain, or the foot starts to swell,*
> ✚TAKE YOUR CHILD TO HOSPITAL

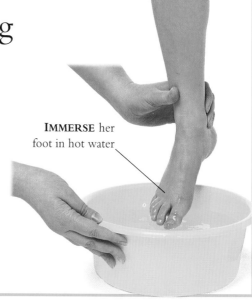

IMMERSE her foot in hot water

SNAKE BITE

Recognising a snake bite
- *A pair of puncture marks*
- *Severe pain, redness, and swelling around bite* • *Vomiting* • *Disturbed vision* • *Breathing difficulties*
- *Increased salivation and sweating*

> **IF** *your child develops ANAPHYLACTIC SHOCK, see p.91.* **IF** *she loses consciousness, see UNCONSCIOUS BABY p.16; CHILD p.22. Be prepared to resuscitate. If breathing, place her in the RECOVERY POSITION.*

HELP her to sit down

1 Help your child to sit or lie down, making sure that the wounded part is *below* the level of her heart.

> **DO NOT** *let your child walk.*
> **DO NOT** *apply a tourniquet, cut out the wound, or try to suck out the venom.*
> *An accurate description of the snake will help doctors treat the injury.*

KEEP injury below level of heart

2 Reassure her. Keep her calm and still to stop the venom spreading through her body. Wash the wound gently with soap and water if available.

93

REASSURE child and keep her still

WASH wound gently with soap and water

PUT padding between limbs

3 Immobilise the injured area using padding and broad- and narrow-fold bandages at knees and ankles (see p.76).

☎ CALL AN AMBULANCE
OR
✚ TAKE YOUR CHILD TO HOSPITAL

TIE broad-fold bandage at knees

TIE narrow-fold bandage around ankles

HYPOTHERMIA

Hypothermia occurs when the body temperature falls. Deep hypothermia, where the body temperature has fallen to a very low level, is extremely dangerous. An older child is most likely to develop hypothermia after over-exertion outside in poor weather conditions, or after falling into very cold water. For babies, see opposite.

GIVE her a warm bath

Recognising hypothermia
• *Shivering* • *Cold, pale, dry skin*
• *Listlessness or confusion* • *Failing consciousness* • *Slow, shallow breathing*
• *Weakening pulse*

1 Give your child a warm bath, if she is able to climb in herself. When her skin colour has returned to normal, help her out, dry her quickly, and wrap her in warm towels or blankets.

WRAP her in warm towels

DRESS her and put her to bed, wrapped in blankets

COVER her head with a hat

WARM her hands with gloves

2 Dress your child with warm clothes and put her to bed, covered with plenty of blankets. Cover her head with a hat and make sure that the room is warm. Stay with her.

☏ CALL A DOCTOR

DO NOT *put a source of direct heat, such as a hot-water bottle, next to the child's skin. The child must warm up gradually.*

94

HELP her to
sip a warm
drink

3 Give your child a warm
drink and some high-energy
foods, such as chocolate. Do not
leave her alone until you are sure
that her colour and temperature
have returned to normal.

> **IF** *your child loses consciousness,*
> *assess her condition (see*
> *UNCONSCIOUS BABY p.16; CHILD*
> *p.22). Be prepared to resuscitate.*
> ☎ CALL AN AMBULANCE

STAY with her until
colour and temperature
have returned to normal

95

Hypothermia in babies

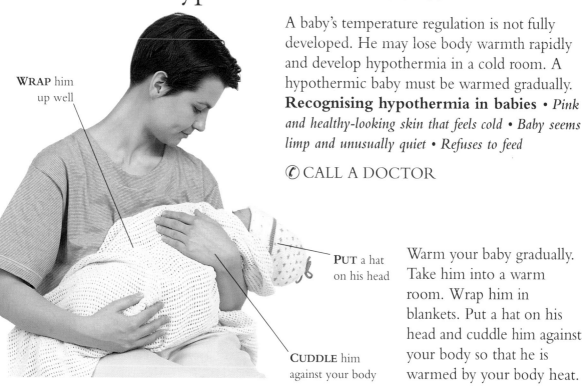

WRAP him
up well

A baby's temperature regulation is not fully
developed. He may lose body warmth rapidly
and develop hypothermia in a cold room. A
hypothermic baby must be warmed gradually.
Recognising hypothermia in babies • *Pink*
and healthy-looking skin that feels cold • *Baby seems*
limp and unusually quiet • *Refuses to feed*

Ⓒ CALL A DOCTOR

PUT a hat
on his head

CUDDLE him
against your body

Warm your baby gradually.
Take him into a warm
room. Wrap him in
blankets. Put a hat on his
head and cuddle him against
your body so that he is
warmed by your body heat.

FROSTBITE

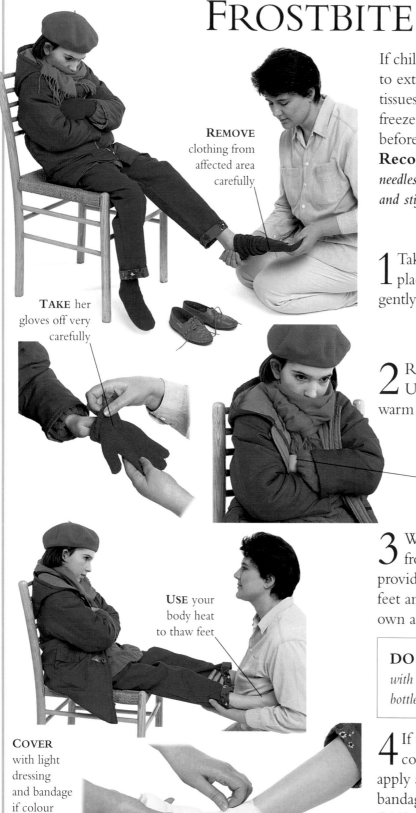

REMOVE clothing from affected area carefully

TAKE her gloves off very carefully

WARM hands with her own body heat, under armpits

USE your body heat to thaw feet

COVER with light dressing and bandage if colour does not return

If children are accidentally exposed to extreme weather conditions, the tissues of the fingers and toes may freeze. Get your child to shelter before you start treatment.
Recognising frostbite • *Pins and needles* • *Numbing* • *Skin feeling hard and stiff, turning white, and waxy*

1 Take your child into a warm place. Sit her down then very gently remove her socks and shoes.

2 Remove gloves and any rings. Undo her coat. Tell her to warm her hands under her armpits.

3 When the feet or toes are frozen, to reduce swelling and provide warmth, raise your child's feet and warm her toes under your own armpits.

> **DO NOT** *warm by rubbing or with direct heat, such as hot-water bottles.* **NEVER** *burst blisters.*

4 If the skin is broken or the colour does not return rapidly, apply a soft gauze dressing and bandage it lightly in place.
✚ TAKE YOUR CHILD TO HOSPITAL

96

HEAT EXHAUSTION

This condition may develop in hot, humid weather and is caused by dehydration. Children who are unwell, particularly with diarrhoea and vomiting, and those not used to playing in the heat are most at risk.

Recognising heat exhaustion • *Headache and dizziness* • *Nausea* • *Sweating* • *Pale, clammy skin* • *Cramps* • *Rapid, weakening pulse*

1 Take your child into the shade or into a cool room. Help him to lie down.

LAY child down in cool room

PUT folded towel or cushion under his head

2 Raise and support your child's legs on some pillows. This improves blood supply to the brain. Encourage him to rest.

RAISE his legs

97

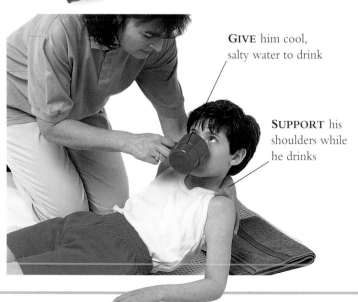

GIVE him cool, salty water to drink

SUPPORT his shoulders while he drinks

3 Help your child to sit up and sip as much cool, salty water (a solution of 5ml/1 teaspoon of salt per litre of fluid) or juice as he can manage. This replaces salt lost from the body.

IF *he loses consciousness, assess his condition (see UNCONSCIOUS BABY p16; CHILD, p.22). Be prepared to resuscitate. If breathing, place him in the RECOVERY POSITION.*

☎ CALL AN AMBULANCE

HEATSTROKE

If the body becomes severely overheated in hot surroundings, heatstroke may occur.

Recognising heatstroke

- *Sudden onset of headache*
- *Confusion* • *Hot, flushed, dry skin* • *Rapid deterioration in level of response* • *A full, bounding pulse* • *Temperature above 40°C (104°F)*

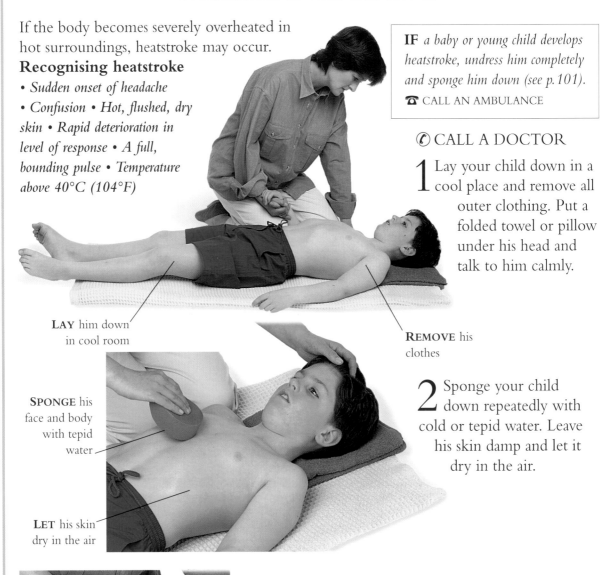

IF *a baby or young child develops heatstroke, undress him completely and sponge him down (see p.101).*
☎ CALL AN AMBULANCE

Ⓒ CALL A DOCTOR

1 Lay your child down in a cool place and remove all outer clothing. Put a folded towel or pillow under his head and talk to him calmly.

LAY him down in cool room

REMOVE his clothes

SPONGE his face and body with tepid water

2 Sponge your child down repeatedly with cold or tepid water. Leave his skin damp and let it dry in the air.

LET his skin dry in the air

COOL him by fanning

3 Fan your child by hand or with an electric fan to bring his temperature down.

IF *he loses consciousness, assess his condition (see UNCONSCIOUS BABY p16; CHILD, p.22). Be prepared to resuscitate. If breathing, place him in the RECOVERY POSITION.*
☎ CALL AN AMBULANCE

SUNBURN

TAKE him into shade

GIVE him cold water to sip

Sunburn is red, itchy, and tender. Babies and young children are particularly vulnerable and should wear a hat and protective cream or clothing in the sun.

IF *there is blistering,* Ⓒ CALL A DOCTOR

1 Move your child into the shade or into a cool room and give him a cold drink.

2 Apply calamine cream or a special after-sun cream to soothe the skin.

IF *your child is restless, flushed, dizzy, has a temperature or headache, see* HEATSTROKE, *opposite.*

APPLY cooling cream to reduce discomfort

99

HEAT RASH

Recognising heat rash • *A prickly, red rash particularly around the sweat glands on the chest and back and under the arms*

Sit your child down in a cool room and undress her. Sponge her down with cool water. Pat her almost dry with a soft towel, leaving the skin slightly damp. Apply calamine cream.

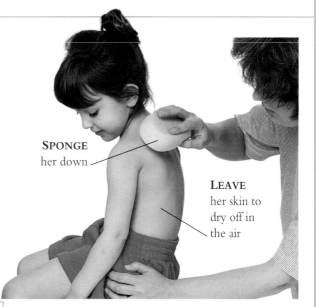

SPONGE her down

LEAVE her skin to dry off in the air

IF *your baby develops heat rash, remove some of her clothes to cool her, or bathe her in tepid water. Dry her gently, leaving her skin slightly damp.*

IF *the rash has not faded after 12 hours, or if her temperature is raised,* Ⓒ CALL A DOCTOR

FEVER

A body temperature that is above the normal level of 37°C (98.6°F) indicates fever. An infection is the usual cause. If your child also has a bad headache, you should study the information on MENINGITIS (see opposite). A moderate fever is not harmful, but a temperature of above 40°C (102°F) can be dangerous, particularly in babies and very young children.

Recognising a fever • *Raised temperature* • *A very pale face and a chilled feeling, with goose pimples* • *Shivering, with chattering teeth*
As the fever advances • *Hot, flushed skin* • *General achiness* • *Sweating* • *Headache*

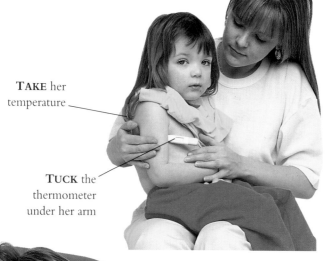

TAKE her temperature

TUCK the thermometer under her arm

1 Lift your child's arm and tuck the pointed end of the thermometer into her armpit. Fold her arm over her chest and leave the thermometer in place for the recommended time. A digital thermometer is the easiest to use.

LAY her down in bed or on the sofa

2 Make your child comfortable on a bed or sofa, but do not cover her. To help bring down her temperature, make sure she has plenty of water or diluted fruit juice to drink.

PROVIDE her with plenty to drink

GIVE her recommended dose of paracetamol syrup

3 You can give your child the recommended dose of paracetamol syrup to help reduce her temperature. If your child is very hot, sponge her down as well, (see opposite).

> **IF** *your baby is under three months old, she should not be given paracetamol syrup, unless you are advised to do so by your doctor.*

100

Cooling babies and young children

In babies and children under four years of age, there is some risk of FEBRILE CONVULSIONS (see p.32). If your child's temperature rises above 40°C (102°F), Ⓒ CALL A DOCTOR.

Babies

Undress your baby down to his nappy and cool him by lightly sponging his body with tepid water. Try to keep him calm.

Young children

Undress your child and cool her by sponging her with tepid water. Continue for up to 30 minutes. Take her temperature again.

UNDRESS him

COOL him by sponging with tepid water

LET his skin dry in the air

> **FEVER** *can also be caused by too much sun, see* HEATSTROKE, *p. 98.*

101

SPONGE her down

LET her skin dry in the air

Meningitis

She may shield her eyes from the light

This is an inflammation of the tissues that surround the brain. It is a very serious condition and must be treated promptly.

Recognising meningitis • *Fever* • *Listlessness* • *Vomiting* • *Loss of appetite* • *Headache or, in babies, a slightly tense fontanelle* • *Pain in eyes from light* • *Pain and stiffness in the neck* • *Convulsions* • *A rash of red or purple blood spots* • *A change for the worse in a child who has recently had an infection*

Make your child comfortable, lying back against pillows or cushions.
Ⓒ CALL A DOCTOR URGENTLY

VOMITING

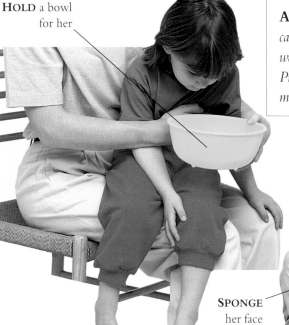

HOLD a bowl for her

> **A BABY** *suffering repeated vomiting and diarrhoea can become dehydrated. Give drinks of cooled, boiled water, but no milk unless you are breast-feeding. Prolonged vomiting may need to be treated with mineral replacement drinks.* ℗ CALL A DOCTOR

1 Hold your child over a bowl or basin. Support her upper body with your free hand while she is being sick. Reassure her.

SPONGE her face gently

2 Once she has stopped vomiting, wipe her face and around her mouth with a sponge or cloth wrung out in tepid water.

GIVE her water to drink

3 Give her drinks of water to replace any fluid loss and to remove the unpleasant taste. Encourage her to sip each drink slowly.

LET her rest

4 Let her rest quietly, in bed if she wants to. Make sure the bowl is still at hand for further sickness attacks, and provide a fresh drink of water.

GIVE her some fresh water

LEAVE a bowl for her

STOMACH ACHE

PROP her up against cushions or pillows

1 Make your child comfortable on a sofa or bed. If she is having difficulty breathing, help her to lie back against cushions or pillows. She may want to be sick so leave a container nearby.

> **IF** *the pain is severe, or does not subside after 30 minutes,*
> ℭ CALL A DOCTOR

2 Warmth may help to relieve the pain. Fill a hot-water bottle – it must be covered – and give it to your child to hold against her stomach. Avoid giving her anything to eat.

PROVIDE a bowl if she feels sick

GIVE her a covered hot-water bottle to hold against her stomach

103

Appendicitis

Inflammation of the appendix is rare under the age of two but may affect older, especially teenage, children.

Recognising appendicitis • *Waves of pain in the middle of the abdomen* • *Acute pain settling in the right lower abdomen* • *Raised temperature* • *Loss of appetite* • *Nausea* • *Vomiting* • *Diarrhoea*

> **APPENDICITIS** *must be treated promptly. Help your child to lie down on a sofa or bed. Do not give him anything to eat or drink.*
> ℭ CALL A DOCTOR

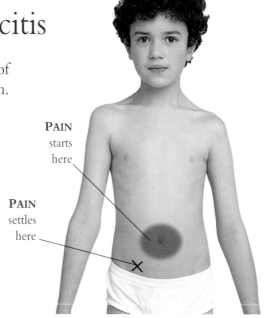

PAIN starts here

PAIN settles here

EARACHE

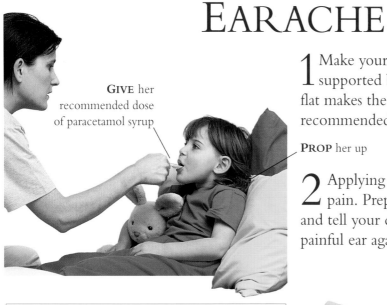

GIVE her recommended dose of paracetamol syrup

1 Make your child comfortable. Sit her up supported by pillows or cushions if lying flat makes the earache worse. Give her the recommended dose of paracetamol syrup.

PROP her up

2 Applying heat may help to soothe the pain. Prepare a covered hot-water bottle and tell your child to lie down with her painful ear against it.

PROVIDE a covered hot-water bottle to hold against her ear

IF *pain does not begin to subside, or if there is a discharge from the ear, fever, or a hearing loss,* ℂ CALL A DOCTOR

Pressure-change earache

This may happen on plane journeys, particularly when taking off or landing, or when travelling through tunnels. To make the ears "pop" so that the pressure is relieved, your child should close her mouth, hold her nose and blow down it. Sucking a sweet may also help.

TELL her to pinch her nose, close her mouth, and "blow" her nose

TOOTHACHE

GIVE her recommended dose of paracetamol syrup

PROVIDE a covered hot-water bottle to lie against

MAKE her comfortable

1 Arrange an early appointment with your child's dentist. Meanwhile, give her the recommended dose of paracetamol syrup to relieve the pain.

2 If lying down does not help to relieve the pain, prop your child up with pillows or cushions. The warmth of a covered hot-water bottle held against the cheek may comfort her.

> **IF** *jaw is swollen and pain is severe,* © CALL A DOCTOR.

CRAMP

STRAIGHTEN her leg

EASE her foot upwards and forwards

SUPPORT her foot in your hand

MASSAGE affected muscles

Cramp is a painful muscle spasm that often affects the foot and calf muscles. You can relieve the pain by massaging and stretching the affected muscles.

1 Help your child to sit down then raise her leg and straighten her knee. Ease her toes upwards to flex the foot.

2 Gently but firmly knead the affected muscle with your fingertips until the spasm has passed completely.

FIRST AID KIT

A well-stocked first aid kit

1 small roller bandage
1 large roller bandage
1 small conforming bandage
1 large conforming bandage
2 eye pads with bandages
Scissors
Calamine cream
Pack of gauze swabs
2 triangular bandages
Hypoallergenic tape
2 sterile pads
Waterproof plasters
1 finger bandage and applicator
Tweezers
1 sterile dressing with bandage

Keep first aid kits in your car and in your home. You can buy ready-made-up standard kits. You may want to add extra dressings and bandages, and disposable gloves. Make sure your first aid box is readily accessible and easy to identify, and check the contents regularly. Don't keep medicines in the first aid box; they should be locked in a medicine cabinet. A well-stocked kit might contain the articles shown below.

Dressings

Plasters (adhesive dressings) are used for minor wounds. Keep several different sizes and shapes. Keep a selection of larger sterile dressings for more serious wounds.

Scissors

Tweezers

Calamine cream or lotion

Plasters

Gauze swabs

Eye pad with bandage

Sterile non-adhesive pad

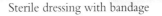

Sterile dressing with bandage

Bandages

Keep a variety of bandages to secure dressings and support injured joints. Conforming bandages shape themselves to the contours of the body and so are easy to use. Triangular bandages can be used as slings and for broad- and narrow-fold bandages.

Hypoallergenic tape for securing dressings

Small conforming bandage

Large conforming bandage

Clip secures bandage

Applicator

Crepe roller bandage

Finger bandage

Large roller bandage

Safety pins

Folded triangular bandage

Other useful items

A variety of household items are invaluable for first aid emergencies. If you don't have exactly the right materials, you can improvise successfully. Keep the following articles to hand.

Flannel

Use a flannel soaked in water to make a cold compress or to sponge a child with a fever.

Sheet and pillow case

A clean cotton sheet or pillowcase makes an excellent loose protective covering for burns.

Kitchen film

Plastic kitchen film can be used to dress burns and seal chest wounds.

Plastic bags

A clean plastic bag can be put over a burned foot or hand and lightly secured with bandages or tape.

107

DRESSINGS

Covering a wound with a dressing will help prevent infection and help the blood-clotting process. Dressings should not be fluffy and need to be large enough to cover the wound and the surrounding area. Always wash your hands before you apply dressings and wear disposable gloves if you have them. If blood soaks through a dressing, place another on top. Make sure any bandages are not too tight, (see opposite).

Plaster

Remove wrapping and, holding the pad over the wound, peel back the protective strips. Press the ends and edges down.

Sterile pad

PLACE non-sticky side over wound

BANDAGE the pad in place

SECURE end of bandage with tape

1 Place the pad shiny side down directly over the wound.

2 Secure the pad with a bandage, working from below the injury up the limb.

3 Secure the end of the bandage with hypoallergenic tape.

Sterile dressing with bandage

PLACE the pad over the wound

WIND the bandage up the limb

TIE ends in a reef knot

1 Hold the bandage either side of the dressing, and place the pad over the wound.

2 Leaving the short end hanging, wind the other end around the limb until the dressing is covered.

3 Tie the two ends of the bandage in a REEF KNOT (see p.76), over the pad.

BANDAGING

Use bandages to secure dressings, to help control bleeding, and to support injuries. Roller bandages can be used for any part of the body; conforming bandages are especially useful for bandaging joints or heads as they mould themselves to the shape of the body.

DO NOT *apply a bandage too tightly – it will impair the circulation. To check, press on your child's nail or a patch of skin, then release pressure. The colour should return rapidly. If it does not, loosen the bandages.*

Roller bandage

SUPPORT the injured limb in your hand

WIND bandage up the limb

SECURE end of bandage with adhesive tape

1 Place the end of the bandage on the arm below the injury and hold the bandage roll in your other hand.

2 Still supporting the injury, wind the bandage around the arm, winding up the limb.

3 Make two straight turns to finish. Secure the end with tape. Check your child's circulation (see above).

109

Hand bandage

MAKE two straight turns around wrist

BANDAGE in a figure-of-eight movement around palm then wrist

FINISHED bandage

SECURE at wrist with tape

1 Supporting the injury, hold the end of the bandage on the wrist and make two straight turns.

2 Take the bandage across the back of the hand to the base of the little finger, then around the palm, and up between the thumb and forefinger, and across the back of the hand to the wrist. Repeat the "figure-of-eight" until the hand is covered.

TRIANGULAR BANDAGES

These are sold singly in sterile packs or can be made from a square of strong fabric folded diagonally in half. Triangular bandages are used for BROAD-FOLD and NARROW-FOLD BANDAGES (see p.76), or slings. Arm slings support injured arms or wrists, or take weight off an injured shoulder. Elevation slings are used for arm and upper body injuries where bleeding, pain, or swelling need to be reduced. (For REEF KNOT see p.76.)

Arm sling

DRAPE long edge of triangle on uninjured side

SUPPORT arm

1 Place the bandage between your child's arm and chest, easing one end up around the back of his neck on the injured side.

TIE a reef knot at shoulder

BRING lower end up over forearm

2 Take the lower end of the bandage up over your child's forearm to the end at the shoulder and tie a REEF KNOT (see p.76) just below the shoulder.

MAKE the reef knot comfortable

TUCK in surplus fabric at elbow

3 Fold in the surplus fabric at the corner near the elbow and pin it to the bandage.

Improvised slings

If your child injures her shoulder, arm, or hand out of doors, you can improvise a sling to support the injury until she receives further treatment.

SUPPORT injury in coat fastening

Undo a coat button and tuck the hand of the injured arm inside the fastening.

PIN sleeve to coat

Alternatively, pin your child's sleeve up on the opposite side of his chest.

110

Elevation sling

REST fingertips on shoulder of uninjured side

HOLD top corner at shoulder

DRAPE long edge across body

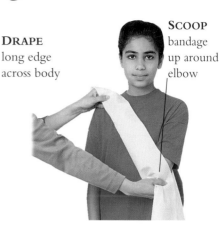

SCOOP bandage up around elbow

1 Bring the arm on the injured side across your child's chest. Ask her to support her elbow.

2 Lay the bandage over your child's arm, with the long edge hanging on the uninjured side. Hold the top corner at the shoulder.

3 Fold long edge of bandage in under injured arm.

TIE ends just in front of shoulder on uninjured side

4 Bring the other end up around her back, holding the elbow securely in the fabric. Tie a REEF KNOT (p.76) just below the shoulder and tuck the ends in.

111

GATHER slack fabric at elbow and tuck in behind

OR

PIN slack fabric to front of sling

5 Secure the bandage by twisting the excess fabric and tucking it in at the elbow. Pin in place.

Finished sling raises, immobilizes, and supports the injury.

SAFETY IN THE HOME

Most accidents occur at home and over half involve children under the age of five. Many accidents are preventable if you:

- Alter the layout and position of objects and furniture at home.
- Make sure windows are closed, or inaccessible.
- Never confuse containers by putting a dangerous substance, such as bleach, in a bottle that used to contain a harmless drink.
- Never tell your child that medicines and pills are special sweeties.
- Check for potential hazards when visiting friends or relatives and ask if you can move sharp or breakable objects.
- Teach your child basic safety rules.

ELECTRICITY

Protect your child from electric shock (see p.12):

- Cover sockets: put heavy furniture in front of them, or fit plastic covers.
- Put only one or two plugs into each socket – overloading can start a fire.
- Wire plugs safely – follow instructions and check that you have the right fuse.
- Check that old flexes are not worn – a child may try to chew protuding wires.
- Tidy up trailing wires
- Unplug electrical appliances at night, particularly the television.
- Fit an RCD (residual current device).

GAS

Find out where your gas tap is in case there is a leak. If you smell gas:

- Don't turn the lights on or off, or use any electric switches – there might be a spark that could cause an explosion.
- Don't light matches or cigarettes.
- Turn off the gas.
- Open the windows.
- Call the gas company.

FIRE

If fire breaks out at home, it could be a matter of minutes before smoke overcomes you.

Fit at least one smoke detector per floor
If your house is on one level, fit a detector between the sitting room and the bedrooms. If your house is on two or more levels, fit one detector at the foot of the stairs and another outside the bedrooms upstairs.

Have an escape plan (see p. 11). Make sure the whole family knows what to do if there is a fire.

Practise a fire drill with your children
- Shout 'fire' • Set off the smoke detector • Tell everyone to drop to the floor and crawl to the exit from the room • Shut the door behind you
- Don't go back for pets or treasured possessions.

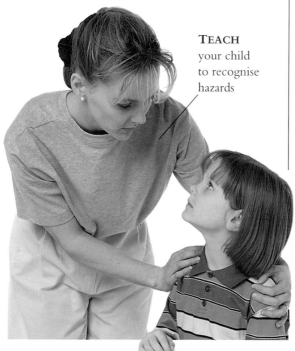

TEACH your child to recognise hazards

> **KEEP** *emergency numbers by the telephone, and make sure the babysitter knows where they are.*

HALL AND STAIRS

The staircase is not a safe place for your child to play (see below).

- Make sure that toys are not left there for you to trip over.
- Put a light in your hall or on the landing in case your child gets up at night. Use a low watt bulb, never cover a lamp with a cloth as the cloth can easily catch fire.
- Don't let your child play on the landings or stairs of a communal area in flats, as the banisters may have large gaps between them.

FRONT DOOR

- Don't leave your front door open.
- Don't let your child answer the door to callers.
- Put the door catch out of reach of small children. If your toddler can reach the catch, fix an additional bolt higher up the door and always keep the door bolted.
- Stick plastic safety film over glass doors. This stops the glass from splintering if it gets broken. Better still, fit toughened or laminated glass.
- Put stickers over the glass to make it more noticeable for young children.

FLOOR

Tiled, polished, or hessian-covered floors can be very slippery for toddlers and running children.

- Put non-slip webbing under rugs.
- Keep hall floors free of toys and clutter.
- Check fitted carpets regularly for holes or loose carpet that might catch a toddler's foot.

STAIRS

A child is not co-ordinated enough to be able to walk downstairs safely until he is at least three years old.

- Fit stair gates at the foot and top of the stairs. Vertical posts on stair gates should be no more than 10cm (4in) apart. A young child can get through a 10cm (4in) gap and fall, or get his head stuck. Always open the gate when you are going upstairs or downstairs. Do not climb over it: your children will learn from you.
- Check your banisters for safety. Make sure the handrail is sturdy and check regularly for loose posts. Posts should be no more than 10cm (4in) apart. Do not let your child use the rails as a climbing frame.
- Check the stair carpet. Loose carpet or worn steps can be a hazard.

113

TEACH him to come downstairs backwards

SUPERVISE your toddler on the stairs

KITCHEN

The kitchen may be the busiest part of your house, where you spend a lot of time with your children. Constant bustle and cooking activities make it a potentially hazardous area.

DOOR
- Cover any glass panels with safety film to stop them shattering or splintering should your toddler run into the door.
- Put some colourful stickers on the glass to alert your child.

FLOOR
- Don't let your child play on the area of floor between you and the work surface or where you could trip over him.
- Avoid bumps and falls by wiping up spills immediately.
- Remove pet food bowls after use and keep that part of the floor scrupulously clean.
- Keep a box for tidying away toys and clutter.

WASTEBINS
- Discourage toddlers from rummaging in the wastebin.
- Put sharp-edged cans and lids or broken glass straight into the dustbin.
- Keep the wastebin in a cupboard with a child-resistant safety catch.

KEEP *a fire blanket in the kitchen for smothering flare-ups. If you want to buy a fire extinguisher, consult your local fire brigade to find out which is the most appropriate type. For more on fires, see p.11 and p.112.*

Babies

CHECK that removable trays have strong clasps

ATTACH a safety harness to the clips on either side of the chair

BOTTLES AND FOOD
- Sterilise all your baby's feeding equipment.
- Don't leave a prepared feed standing at room temperature, and don't keep the remains of the last feed. Warmed or reheated feeds are breeding grounds for bacteria that might upset your baby's stomach.

HIGHCHAIRS
- Always use a safety harness.
- Never leave the chair where your baby can reach out and pull objects down from a surface. Keep him amused with a safe toy.
- Never leave your child unattended.

PLAY
- Have a safe area or a playpen where your baby can play and watch you.
- Keep him out of range of any spills from the cooker.

CHOOSE a stable highchair with widely spaced legs.

TABLES AND WORK SURFACES

- Always be aware of your child's reach and keep all heavy, breakable, or sharp objects well back from the edges of surfaces.
- Keep stools or chairs away from tables and work surfaces to prevent your child climbing up on them.
- Tuck flexes of kettles, toasters, blenders, and irons out of reach. Choose a curly flex for your kettle if possible. It is not only boiling, steaming kettles that pose a hazard: water is still hot enough to scald 15 minutes after boiling.
- Leave electrical appliances unplugged when they are not in use.
- Avoid using a tablecloth. It is tempting for a crawling baby or toddler to use it to pull himself up, bringing anything on the table down upon his head. Use table mats instead, or secure the cloth with clips.

CUPBOARDS AND DRAWERS

- Put safety catches on cupboards and drawers particularly those that contain: knives, scissors, and cutlery; heavy pots, pans, or china; dried food, such as lentils or pasta, that may be a choking hazard; alcohol and bottles; medicines, including vitamins; cleaning materials, such as washing powder or bleach, including those with "child-resistant" lids.

FRIDGE

Food poisoning can be caused by poor food storage. Take precautions to minimise risks:

- Keep cooked meat and poultry on a separate shelf from uncooked meat. Cover uncooked meat with kitchen film.
- Don't store food in open tins; tip leftovers into a clean container and put in the fridge.
- Check food regularly, to see that nothing is kept beyond the "sell-by" date.

COOKER

Your child is obviously at risk of burns and scalds from hot fat or boiling water when you are preparing food.

- You can buy safety guards, but remember that a child can still poke fingers through them and be burnt by hot hobs or gas rings.
- Always keep your child away from oven doors; they can get very hot while the oven is in use and will stay hot for some time afterwards. A crawling baby or toddler is particularly at risk. Try to teach your child what "hot" means, so he understands a warning.
- Keep matches well out of reach in a cupboard with a safety catch.

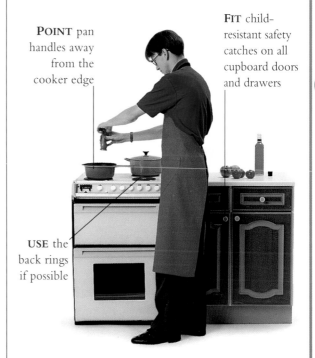

POINT pan handles away from the cooker edge

FIT child-resistant safety catches on all cupboard doors and drawers

USE the back rings if possible

WASHING MACHINE AND TUMBLE DRIER

- Keep small hands away from the glass door. It may get hot while the machine is on.
- Ensure the door is closed while the machine is not in use. Your toddler may try to climb inside, or fill it with toys.

SITTING ROOM

While your children are very young, try to arrange the room so that both children and your valuables are kept out of harm's way. If you have a balcony, block up gaps in the railings with hardboard and check that your child can't climb over. Never leave toys on a high surface as he may attempt to retrieve them.

CARPETS AND CURTAINS
- Check that there are no areas of carpet or rug that have holes or turned up edges; either you or your child could trip up.
- Wind up and tuck away curtain ties and cords for blinds. Children can be strangled if they get caught in dangling cords.

FIREPLACES AND HEATERS
- Don't leave matches or firelighters where your child can reach them.
- Use a fireguard over an open fire. Fix it to the wall to prevent your child pulling it over. Put a guard over gas heaters.
- Never use the fireguard as a shelf or clothes airer.
- Use a spark-guard as well as a fireguard for open fires as an additional precaution.

TELEVISIONS, VIDEOS, AND HI-FI EQUIPMENT
- Fix wiring to the skirting board.
- Run long flexes behind furniture, so that your child won't trip or pull on them.
- Cover any unused plug sockets with plastic safety covers.
- Check that old flexes are not worn.

POSITION electrical equipment against the wall so that your child can't get at the back

SURFACES AND FURNITURE
- Place houseplants out of reach of young children. Some houseplants are poisonous, and others can scratch or produce allergic reactions if touched.
- Keep breakable or heavy objects off low tables and well back from the edges of surfaces such as window sills or mantelpieces.
- Remove glass-topped tables and put corner protectors on sharp table corners.
- Don't leave hot drinks, alcohol, glasses, cigarettes, matches, or lighters on low surfaces, such as coffee tables, where your child can reach them.
  - Keep alcohol in a locked cupboard.
  - Never leave a cigarette burning on the arm of a sofa or armchair. Old foam furniture can be lethal in a fire as it releases toxic fumes within seconds of catching alight.

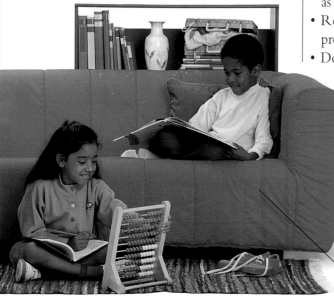

CHOOSE sofas and armchairs with fire-resistant fillings and coverings

TOYS AND PLAYTHINGS

When you buy toys or equipment for your child, follow these guidelines:

- Buy toys that display the appropriate safety mark and buy from a reputable source.
- Make sure that there are no sharp edges, and avoid anything made of thin, rigid plastic.
- Buy non-toxic paints or crayons.
- Don't buy your child second-hand toys that may be covered in paint containing lead.
- Avoid novelty toys that are not designed to be played with by young children: look out for warnings on the packaging.

CHECK that sets of building blocks don't have small pieces that could be a choking hazard for your child

CARING FOR TOYS

- Check toys regularly and throw away any broken ones.
- Don't mix batteries – change them all at the same time, otherwise the strong batteries will make the weak ones very hot.
- Keep toys in a toy box. Toys can bring about accidents or injuries by being left on the floor .

GIVE your child non-toxic paints and crayons

117

Babies and toddlers

- Remove ribbons from a baby's soft toys.
- Check that the eyes, noses, ears, or bells on soft toys and dolls are well secured.
- Attach cot toys with a very short string.
- Remove activity centres or bulky toys from a cot as soon as your child can stand, as they provide a foothold for climbing out.
- Don't let babies chew on furry toys: the fur is a choking hazard for children under one year old.
- Never give a small child a toy that is not recommended for his age-group as it may contain small pieces on which he could choke.
- Always supervise a baby or toddler while he is playing.

MAKE SURE that toys that increase mobility are stable

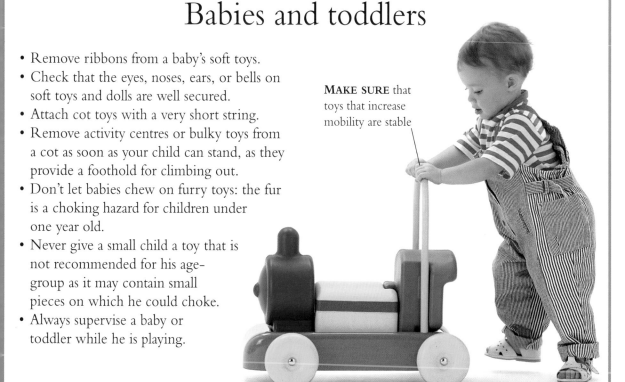

BEDROOMS

The cupboards and drawers in bedrooms are always exciting places for toddlers and young children. Make sure any potentially hazardous items are out of reach, as you may not always know when your child will decide to go exploring on his own.

Babies

COT

- Make sure the cot is deep enough to prevent your baby from climbing out – at least 50cm (1ft 8in) from the top of the mattress to the top of the cot.
- Bar spaces must be between 2.5–6cm (1–2½in) wide to prevent your baby's head being trapped.

- The mattress must be the right size with a gap no larger than 3cm (1½in) around the side. Otherwise the baby's head could get trapped between the side of the cot and the mattress.
- Do not use a pillow for a baby under a year: it could suffocate him. If you need to raise his head, put a pillow underneath the mattress.
- Use a sheet and cellular blankets, rather than a duvet, until your baby is a year old. Your baby may get overheated or kick the duvet over his face and suffocate.
- Always put your baby to sleep on his back or side (never on his front) to lessen risk of cot death.
- Remove bumpers as soon as the baby can sit up – he could use them to climb out.
- Once he starts trying to climb out of the cot, transfer him to a bed. You can fit a bed guard at first, until he is used to the bed.

CHECK the cot dropside has strong clasps that your baby cannot open

ENSURE that bumpers have very short ties, to prevent strangulation

CHANGING AREA

- Keep all changing equipment in one area, so that you never have to leave your baby alone. He will be safest on the floor, but if you have a changing table, remember that he might roll off if left for even a moment.
- Do not have shelves above the changing area in case something falls off.
- Keep mobiles out of his reach.
- If you use talcum powder, sprinkle it on your hands and rub them together to avoid creating a cloud of dust around your baby.

CHANGE your baby on a changing mat on the floor so that he cannot fall

118

Your child's room

BEDS

- Use a bed guard when your toddler first moves to a bed.
- Top bunk beds must have safety rails on both sides and any gaps in the railings or between the top of the mattress and the bottom of the safety rail should be 6–7.5cm (2½–3in).
- A top bunk is not recommended for children under the age of six.
- Never let young children play on the top bunk.
- Move toys from the floor by the bed at night.

AVOID feather pillows and duvets as they can provoke allergies

WINDOWS

Make sure your child can't climb out. Even if his room is on the ground floor, he is in danger if he falls.

- Fix a safety catch, but make sure the window can be opened easily in the event of a fire.
- Try not to place a piece of furniture below a window – it may encourage your child to climb up.

TOYS (see p. 117).

- Try to keep toys with small pieces separate from others, so that you can easily remove them and put them out of reach for a while if your child is sharing a room with a toddler, or if you have young visitors.

PUT non-slip webbing under rugs

119

Your room

- **Medicines and pills** Do not keep them beside your bed or on a dressing table. Put them out of sight and out of reach.
- **Scissors and sewing equipment** Keep these in a drawer or cupboard where your child cannot reach them.
- **Perfume, hairspray, and makeup** These can be harmful if sprayed or rubbed in the eyes, or drunk, so keep them out of reach, or in a drawer with a safety catch.
- **China cups and glasses** Never leave a china cup or a glass on the floor by your bed. If your child is sleeping in your bed at night and rolls out onto the cup or the glass, he could have a serious accident.

BATHROOM

Your child may be at risk from falls, or drowning, or poisoning in the bathroom. Keep the bathroom door shut at all times to discourage him from going in. On the inside of the door, fix the bolt high up, to prevent a small child locking himself in.

SHOWER
- Keep a constant check on the temperature of the water.
- Use non-slip mats in the shower and on the bathroom floor.
- Put safety film on a glass shower door so that glass is held in place in case of an accident.

BATH
- Always check the temperature of the water before your child gets in. A young child can be badly scalded by hot bath water.
- Use non-slip mats in the bath and on the floor by the bath.
- Never leave a young child or baby alone in the bath. A baby can drown in just 2.5cm (1in) of water. If you need to answer the doorbell or telephone, take your child with you.

CUPBOARDS AND CABINETS
- Store bathroom chemicals and other potential poisons, such as toilet cleaners and bleach, out of reach in a cupboard with a safety catch.
- Keep other hazards, such as make-up, aftershave, razors, nail scissors, and any medicines or glass containers, out of reach in a locked medicine cabinet.

TOILET
- Use a special child toilet seat adaptor and step for toddlers, so that they can keep their balance more easily and so feel more secure.
- Keep the toilet seat closed.
- Don't use block toilet cleaners that a small child could pull out and chew.
- Never mix toilet cleaners with bleach as this can give off toxic fumes.
- If your toddler uses a potty, keep it clean, but never leave bleach or cleaning agents inside it.

BATH him away from the tap end

NEVER leave your child unattended in the bath

USE a non-slip mat in the bath

GARDEN

You don't have to be a keen gardener to make your garden into a safe and interesting place for your children to play. Children will find their own corners to play in but you should remove obvious hazards:

- Clear away any rubbish or rubble.

- Check garden furniture or play equipment regularly to make sure that it is stable and safe.
- Keep pets off areas where children play.
- Make sure paving is even and remove moss. Children may easily trip or slip.
- Lock gates that lead out of the garden and make sure fences are secure.

WARN your child not to eat berries or leaves

PLANTS

Many plants are poisonous if eaten and digested in large quantities. Small pieces, or one or two berries, are not fatal, but may cause some discomfort and stomach upset.

- Tell your child about the dangers of eating berries and keep babies and toddlers away from them.
- Remove plants that you know to be poisonous, such as deadly nightshade, laburnum, and toadstools.
- Cut back any prickly plants, such as roses, brambles, and holly – they can give nasty scratches, especially to the eyes.

SUPERVISE your toddler at all times. Check that he is playing in a clean, safe area with safe toys

SHEDS

These are exciting dens for children.

- If your shed is full of gardening equipment or tools, tell your child that it is out of bounds and keep it locked.
- Put any chemicals, such as weedkiller or slug pellets, out of reach.

PONDS, PADDLING POOLS, AND WATER BUTTS

Children are in danger if they slip and fall, even in shallow water.

- Never leave children unattended when they are playing in, or near, water.
- Cover ponds, water butts, and empty dustbins that collect rainwater.
- Always empty out a paddling pool when the children have finished playing in it.

GARDENING

- Don't put down chemicals when children will be playing in the garden.
- Don't mow the lawn while children are close by, as stone chips may be dislodged and fly up into their eyes.
- Fit circuit breakers on all electrical equipment such as mowers and hedge trimmers.
- Put away all garden tools when you have finished using them.

121

OUT AND ABOUT

After the home, most accidents to children occur on the street. Teach your child the rules of the road from an early age, reminding him to stay alert for traffic and to cross in a safe place. It takes a long time for children to develop a true road sense.

BY THE ROAD

- Three-year-olds can learn that the pavement is safe and the road is dangerous.
- Five-year-olds can learn how to cross the road, but they are still not able to put this knowledge into practice on their own.
- Eight-year-olds can cross quiet streets on their own, but are not yet able to judge the speed and distance of traffic.
- Twelve-year-olds can judge the speed of an oncoming car, but are still easily distracted by friends.

IN THE STREET

Whenever you are out with your child, show him how to be aware of his own safety.

- Use reins or a wrist strap for a toddler, to stop him running off.
- Hold a child's hand when you are near the road, or waiting to cross.
- Teach your child by your example and always find a safe place to cross. This may be:

  ▲ *A zebra crossing – wait at the island halfway, if there is one.*

  ▲ *A pelican crossing at traffic lights. Encourage your child to press the button and tell him to wait until the traffic has stopped.*

  ▲ *An underpass.*

  ▲ *A footbridge.*

  ▲ *A large gap between parked cars, where your child can see a long way in both directions.*

Crossing the road

Teach your child the rules of the road.

▲ *Find a safe place to cross, then stop.*

▲ *Stand on the pavement, near the kerb.*

▲ *Look all round for traffic, and listen.*

▲ *If traffic is coming, let it pass.*

▲ *When there is no traffic near, walk straight across the road.*

▲ *Keep looking and listening for traffic while you cross.*

BIKES

- Children younger than 11 years old should not cycle on roads in traffic.
- Arrange for your child to have cycle training before he starts on the roads.
- Make sure your child can be seen when he's riding his bike – with bright fluorescent colours by day and reflectors on his clothes and bike by night. He should have an approved helmet to protect his head.

INSIST he always wears a protective helmet

MAINTAIN the bike in good working order

PLAYING

What may seem common sense to you, is not always obvious to children.

- Teach your child the dangers of playing in open areas such as roads, building sites, and quarries.
- Tell your child not to play in the street, or on a pavement near the kerb.
- Tell him that he must never chase a ball, a pet, or another child into the road.
- Tell him not to try to cross the road from between two closely parked cars.

PRAMS AND BUGGIES

- Never push a pram or buggy out into the traffic – pull it to one side and check whether it is safe to cross. Remember that a buggy sticks out in front of you by at least 1 metre (3 ft).
- When you park a pram or buggy, put on the brakes and point it away from traffic.
- Never tie your dog to the pram.
- Never leave a baby unattended.

HARNESS your baby into his pram

In the playground

Playgrounds should comply with safety standards and recommendations.

- The play area must be safely fenced off, away from roads.
- There should be a soft, even surface, such as bark chippings or rubber tiles around equipment.
- Slides should be no higher than 2.4m (8ft) and preferably constructed on an earth mound to break any falls.
- Roundabouts should be low, with a smooth surface, designed so that children can't get their feet stuck underneath.
- Climbing frames should be no higher than 2.4m (8ft), be completely stable and built over sand or a very soft surface to break falls.
- There should be a clearly defined area for toddlers and young children, set away from the more boisterous activities of older children.
- There should be someone to contact if equipment is faulty.
- Dogs must not be allowed inside.

CHECK that swings are set apart from main play equipment, or fenced off, to prevent children running in front of, or behind, them

MAKE SURE your child is wearing suitable clothing

TEACH your child how to use equipment properly

STRANGERS *Remind your child of the dangers of talking to strangers. Have a code word that a friend can use if meeting your child. Tell your child not to go with anybody unless they use the code.*

GARAGE & CAR SAFETY

GARAGE

- Keep the garage locked and discourage your child from going in there.
- Keep equipment, chemicals, or tools out of your child's reach and locked away, if possible.
- Make sure you know where your child is when you are driving into, or out of, the garage.
- If you keep a freezer in the garage, it should be locked at all times.

CAR

- Never leave a young child unattended in a car.
- Don't let your child play with the window, whether manual or electric. Electric windows can trap a child's head or fingers.
- Remove the cigarette lighter.
- Watch out for your child's fingers when you shut the doors.
- Use child locks on rear doors until your child is at least six years old.
- Teach your child to get out of the car on the pavement side.
- If your child is helping you as you wash or tidy the car, make sure you have removed the keys from the ignition.

CAR SEATS

Always put your child into a special safety seat when you strap him into the car. If you are buying a second-hand car seat, you must buy one that has a known history. Some car seats are reconditioned after a crash and will not be safe. Choose the right seat for the age of your child.

- **Babies** up to 10kg (22lb) – about nine months – should travel in a rear-facing car seat. The baby is harnessed into the seat and the seat is held in place by the car seat belts. You can put this seat on the front passenger seat as the baby's head and back have some protection from a front impact. Your baby will be able to see you as you drive and is less likely to become upset from loss of contact with you.
- Never carry a baby on your lap, or inside your own seatbelt: he would be crushed in a crash.
- **Older babies and toddlers**, up to 18kg (40lb), need a moulded car seat in the back. Some of these seats have an integral harness for the child that fits over his shoulders and between his legs. These seats are kept in place by the adult seat belt, or by straps that you can fix into the car. Other seats use the adult belt to hold both child and seat into the car.
- **Primary school children** (from four or five years old up to 11 years old) should travel in a booster seat. Without it, adult seat belts are neither comfortable nor safe. The shoulder part cuts across the child's neck and the lap strap lies across his stomach. In a crash, the lap strap can damage his liver or spleen. A booster seat raises a young child so the shoulder part lies across his upper chest and the lap strap lies across his hips. A lap strap on its own is not sufficient as it does not restrain the child's upper body.

FIT a moulded car seat for maximum protection

INDEX

Acknowledgments

British Red Cross
First Aid Training Department:
Mr Anthony Kemp, Miss Lyn Covey
Mr Joe Mulligan

Safety in the home: advice on content, and text read by Dr Sara Levene of the Child Accident Prevention Trust

Dorling Kindersley would like to thank:

Lorna Damms and Ros Fishel for editorial help; Sarah Ashun and Gary Ombler for assisting the photographers; Wendy Holmes for makeup; Hilary Bird for the index; the following for modelling:

Children Aleena Awan (4), Navaz Awan (3), Amy Davies (9), Thomas Davies (7), James Dow (6), Kyla Edwards (6), Austin Enil (5), Lia Foa (11), Maya Foa (9), Kashi Gorton (7), Emily Gorton (4), Thomas Greene (5), Alexander Harrison (7), Rupert Harrison (5), Ben Harrison (2), Jessica Harris-Voss (3), Jake Hutton (3 months), Rosemary Kaloki (10), Winnie Kaloki (8), Ella Kaye (11), Maddy Kaye (9), Jade Lamb (3), Emily Leney (5), Harriet Lord (3), Ailsa McCaughrean (4), Fiona Maine (9), Tom Maine (6), Maija Marsh (4), Oliver Metcalf (4), Eloise Morgan (3), Tom Razazan (9), Jimmy Razazan (7), Rebecca Sharples (8), Ben Sharples (6), Thomas Sharples (4), Ben Walker (10), Robyn Walker (8), Amy Beth Walton Evans (2), Hanna Warren-Green (5), Simon Weekes (6), Joseph Weir (2)

Adults Shaila Awan, Georgina Davies, Marion Davies, Sophie Dow, Tina Edwards, Rachel Fitchett, Emma Foa, Caroline Greene, Claire le Bas, Susan Harrison, Victoria Harrison, Julia Harris-Voss, Emma Hutton, Helga Lien Evans, Sylvie Jordan, Jane Kaloki, David Kaye, Louise Kaye, Geraldine McCaughrean, Diana Maine, Brian Marsh, Jonathon Metcalf, Francoise Morgan, Hossein Razazan, Angela Sharples, John Sharples, Vanessa Walker, Catherine Warren-Green, Toni Weekes.

Make-up: Pebbles, Geoff Portas

Additional photographs
Dave King, Ray Mollers, Suzannah Price, Dave Rudkin, Steve Shott

EMERGENCY TELEPHONE NUMBERS

IN AN EMERGENCY GO TO THE NEAREST
TELEPHONE AND DIAL 999. ASK FOR THE
POLICE, AMBULANCE OR FIRE BRIGADE

DOCTOR
Name:
Address:

Telephone:
Surgery Hours:

HEALTH VISITOR
Name:
Clinic Address:

Telephone:
Clinic Hours:

DENTIST
Name:
Address:

Telephone:
Surgery Hours:

HOSPITAL ACCIDENT & EMERGENCY
Address:

Telephone:

LATE NIGHT CHEMIST
Address:

LOCAL POLICE STATION
Address:

Telephone:

GAS EMERGENCY SERVICE
Telephone:

ELECTRICITY EMERGENCY SERVICE
Telephone:

WATER EMERGENCY SERVICE
Telephone:

TAXI
Telephone:

**IN CASE OF AN EMERGENCY
PLEASE CALL:**

British Red Cross

The British Red Cross runs first aid courses for all ages.
For further information, get in touch with your local
Branch Headquarters; you will find the number in the
telephone directory or in the Yellow Pages.

**National Headquarters
British Red Cross**
9 Grosvenor Crescent
London SW1X 7EJ
071-235 5454

*Details of the royalties
payable to the British Red
Cross Society can be obtained
by writing to the publisher
Dorling Kindersley at the
following address: 9 Henrietta
Street, London WC2E 8PS*

128